Bioceramics: Materials and Applications III

Related titles published by The American Ceramic Society:

Surface Active Materials (Ceramic Transactions Volume 101)
Edited by David E. Clark, Joseph Simmons, and Catherine Simmons
©2000, ISBN 1-57498-079-3

Bioceramics: Materials and Applications II (Ceramic Transactions Volume 63)
Edited by Richard P. Rusin and Gary S. Fischman
©1996, ISBN: 1-57498-006-8

Bioceramics: Materials and Applications (Ceramic Transactions Volume 48)
Edited by Gary Fischman, Alexis Clare, and Larry Hench
©1995, ISBN: 0-944904-82-3

For information on ordering titles published by The American Ceramic Society, or to request a publications catalog, please contact our Customer Service Department at 614-794-5890 (phone), 614-794-5892 (fax),<customersrvc@acers.org> (e-mail), or write to Customer Service Department, 735 Ceramic Place, Westerville, OH 43081, USA.

Visit our on-line book catalog at <www.ceramics.org>.

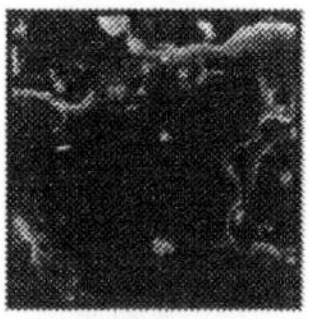

Ceramic Transactions
Volume 110

Bioceramics: Materials and Applications III

Edited by

Laurie George
American Dental Association Health Foundation

Richard P. Rusin
3M Corporation

Gary S. Fischman
University of Illinois

Vic Janas
Johnson & Johnson

Published by

The American Ceramic Society
735 Ceramic Place
Westerville, Ohio 43081

Proceedings of the Bioceramics: Materials and Applications symposium, held at the 101st Annual Meeting of The American Ceramic Society, Indianapolis, Indiana, April 25–28, 1999.

COVER PHOTO: "Ca-phosphate coating applied to the surface of zirconia ceramics by plasma coating," is courtesy of J. Cihlar, M. Jez, K Castkova, and M. Trunec, and appears as figure 3 in their paper "Oxide Ceramics with Calcium Phosphate Coatings," which begins on page 157.

Library of Congress Cataloging-in-Publication Data
A CIP record for this book is available from the Library of Congress.

For information on ordering titles published by The American Ceramic Society, or to request a publications catalog, please call 614-794-5890.

4 3 2 1–03 02 01 00

ISSN 1042-1122
ISBN 1-57498-102-1

Contents

Preface viii

In Vitro Stability Predictions for the Bone/Bioglass and Bone/HA Interactions 1
Melissa J. Crimp, Dean A. Oppermann, and Udhav U. Doctor

Glass-Hydroxyapatite Coatings on Titanium-Based Implants 15
J.M. Gomez-Vega, E. Saiz, and A.P. Tomsia, G.W. Marshall, and S.J. Marshall

Synthesis of Hydroxyapatite via Mechanical Activation 25
K.C.B. Yeong, J. Wang, and S.C. Ng

Preparation of Biomimetic HA Precursors at 37°C in Urea- and Enzyme Urease-Containing Synthetic Body Fluids 39
Defne Bayraktar and A. Cüneyt Tas

Physical Characteristics of Sintered Hydroxyapatite 53
T.P. Hoepfner and E.D. Case

Spray Dried Titania Cell Carriers 67
K.-L. Eckert, E. Wintermantel, and R. Gadow

Crystallization of SiC on Biological Carbon Precursors 81
H. Sieber, H. Friedrich, A. Kaindl, and P. Greil

Surface Properties of Layered Double Hydroxide Nanocomposites 93
O.C. Wilson Jr., T. Olorunyolemi, A. Jaworski, L. Borum, D. Young, E. Dickens, and C. Oriakhi

Near-Net-Shape Forming Technique for Bioceramic Components 103
A. Salomoni, I. Stamenkovic, L. Esposito, and A. Tucci

In Vitro Bioresorbable Fiber Dissolution 113
S.H. Lee and A.G. Clare

Scope of Piezoelectric Devices in Determining Inner Ear Function 129
N. Mukherjee, R.D. Roseman, and J.P. Willging

Characterization of Plasma Sprayed HA/ZrO_2 Composite Coatings 145
L. Fu, K.A. Khor, V.J.P. Lim

Oxide Ceramics with Calcium Phosphate Coatings 157
J. Cihlar, M. Jez, K. Castkova, and M. Trunec

Processing, Biocompatibility and Biomechanical Testing of Porous Alumina Ceramics 167
Susmita Bose, Jens Darsell, Lihua Yang, Dipak K. Sarkar, and Amit Bandyopadhyay

Development of Bioceramic Tissue Scaffold via Fused Deposition of Ceramics 183
Iván A. Cornejo, Thomas F. McNulty, Shelliam Lee, Ernest Bianchi, Stephen C. Danforth, Ahmad Safari, Kevor S. TenHuisen, and Victor F. Janas

Index 197

Preface

This symposium on bioceramics is the seventh in a series that looks at biomedical materials from a ceramics perspective. This symposium was sponsored by NICE and the Engineering Ceramics and Glass and Optical Materials divisions of The American Ceramic Society. The program was held at the 101st Annual Meeting of The American Ceramic Society in Indianapolis, Indiana, April 25–28, 1999, under the title "Bioceramics: Materials and Applications." Fifty-seven oral and poster presentations were made.

Laurie George
Richard P. Rusin
Gary S. Fischman
Vic Janas

IN VITRO STABILITY PREDICTIONS FOR THE BONE/BIOGLASS AND BONE/HA INTERACTIONS

Melissa J. Crimp, Dean A. Oppermann, and Udhav U. Doctor
Department of Materials Science & Mechanics
Michigan State University
East Lansing, MI 48824-1226

ABSTRACT

Electroacoustic measurements of the zeta (ζ) potential as a function of pH were collected and used to probe the nature of ionic contributions on the bond formed between bone and 2 types of Bioglass (45S5 and 52S) and bone and hydroxyapatite (HA). Powders of each of the synthetic materials and wet bone were dispersed into an electrolyte solution comprised of physiologic saline (0.154M NaCl), electroacoustic measurements collected, and the ζ-potential calculated as a function of pH. The ζ-potential and particle size were then used to calculate the stability of the composite dispersion, where stability is the ability of a particulate to remain in suspension unagglomerated. These stability values were then used to predict the homo- (synthetic to synthetic and bone to bone) versus heterocoagulation (synthetic to bone) behaviors for these synthetic/bone systems. *Single* component suspensions of bone and each of the synthetic materials demonstrated stability against agglomeration. Stability calculations predict that the 45S5/bone interaction was unstable for the pH range tested (5-9), the 52S/bone interaction was stable in the same pH range and the HA/bone interaction was unstable in the pH range, including pH 7.4, the normal *in vivo* pH. These results establish one factor responsible for the observed physicochemical bonding between bone and 45S5 Bioglass and bone/HA noted by many in the orthopedic community. In addition, from the standpoint of ionic attraction, the 52S Bioglass/bone system is not as suitable in terms of bonding to bone in comparison to the 45S5 Bioglass/bone system.

INTRODUCTION

Recent advancements in biomaterials technology have resulted from development of surface reactive or bioactive ceramics. Properties and uses for glass-ceramics have been widely documented[1-6], focusing on the glass ceramics such as Bioglass and on calcium phosphate ceramics such as hydroxyapatite (HA) and BCP (Biphasic Calcium Phosphate)[7,8]. These materials are commonly used as coatings for implants or in bone replacement applications and are characterized by their ability to achieve a strong interfacial bond between implant and bone.

Even though excellent bonding of both Bioglass and HA to bone has been well-documented[9,10], the mechanisms for this bonding are not completely understood. One explanation of HA's ability to bond to bone is that calcium phosphates such as HA have been shown to be water soluble, containing the same apatite crystal chemistry as the mineral portion of bone. HA dissolves in physiologic solution, re-precipitates on the bone surface, exhibiting epitaxial growth[9]. This leads to the formation of a granular bonding layer between bone and HA[11]. However, this explanation assumes intimate contact between the HA and the bone upon HA re-precipitation. It is the researchers opinion that this contact and therefore bonding is enhanced by the *in vivo* ionic activity of the HA particles and bone.

Hench attributes the bonding between Bioglasses and bone to kinetic modification of the surface that occurs upon implantation[12]. This kinetic modification leads to the formation of a bioactive hydroxylcarbonate (HCA) layer that is structurally and chemically equivalent to the mineral phase of bone. Hench has shown that the collagenous constituent of soft tissues can strongly adhere to Bioglasses. The collagen fibrils are woven into the interface by growth of the HCA layer. The HCA/collagen interface thickness mimics that of tendons and ligaments to bone. Even though the mechanisms for the HCA formation have been well documented the mechanisms for collagen adhesion are not completely understood.

The degree of ionic activity between bone and synthetic materials may be assessed through the zeta (ζ) potential as calculated from the acoustophoretic particle mobility. O'Brien [13,14] and Oja[15] have extensively described the electrokinetic phenomena of acoustophoresis. Particles suspended in an electrolyte generate an acoustic wave when subjected to an alternating electric field due to any surface charge and density differential between the particles and the liquid ($\Delta\rho$). This acoustic wave is measured as pressure amplitude per unit of applied electric field ($ESA(\omega)$) from which the particle dynamic mobility ($\mu_d(\omega)$) is calculated using an equation derived by O'Brien[13,14]:

$$\mu_d(\omega) = ESA(\omega) / \phi\Delta\rho c \qquad (1)$$

where ϕ is the volume fraction solid and c is the velocity of sound in the suspension. The ζ-potential is calculated using the acoustophoretic mobility with a correction for the particle inertia $G(\alpha)^{-1}$, in an alternating field. This correction reduces the velocity amplitude of particle motion. The equation to calculate the ζ-potential was derived using the Helmholtz-Smoluchowski equation [13,14]:

$$\zeta = (\mu\eta / \varepsilon_o \varepsilon_r) G(\alpha)^{-1} \quad (2)$$

Where ε_o is the permitivity in a vacuum, ε_r is the relative permitivity, and $G(\alpha)^{-1}$ is given by:

$$G(\alpha)^{-1} = \left[1 - \frac{i\alpha(3 + 2\Delta\rho / \rho)}{9\{1 + (1 - i)(\alpha / 2)^{1/2}\}} \right]. \quad (3)$$

Colloidal theory has been used extensively in manufacturing ceramics to eliminate agglomeration and segregation[16-20] of system components such as second phase reinforcements. Van der Waals, steric, and repulsive forces act on colloidal particles (particle size $\leq$ 1μm) to generate either an agglomerated state or a dispersed suspension according to Derjaguin and Landau[21], and Verwey and Overbeek[22] (DLVO) predictions. To describe the effects of homo- and heterocoagulation and to generate a quantitative theory for the overall kinetic stability of a system of non-identical particles, Hogg et al.[23] developed an expression for interparticle stability (W_{ij}). This factor, termed the stability ratio is in effect, the ratio of particle collision to collisions that result in agglomeration.

$$W_{ij} = \int_{a_i + a_j}^{\infty} \exp\left(\frac{V_T}{kT}\right) \frac{dr}{r^2} \quad (4)$$

In Equation 4, the interparticle stability varies exponentially with the total force, V_T, (attractive and repulsive) and inversely with the square of the particle separation distance, r, from a separation equal to the sum of the two particle radii, a_i and a_j to an infinite separation distance into the solution. The repulsive force, which acts as a barrier to coagulation is proportional to the surface charge of the particle[24]. However, this surface charge is not readily measurable because of continuous ion activity at the particle/fluid interface. Therefore, the surface charge is estimated at the double layer by the ζ-potential which in this study, is measured using electroacoustic (ESA) methods.

EXPERIMENTAL PROCEDURE

Materials

45S5 and 52S Bioglass[1] were used in this study. The Bioglass compositions are given in Table I. The Bioglasses were ground using mortar and pestle and ball milled dry for 48 hours using alumina grinding media prior to ζ-potential measurement.

Stoichiometric HA (Ca/P=1.67) powder was used for this study, with a manufacturers[2] reported particle size of 25 μm. Each of these powders were subsequently ground using mortar and pestle and wet sieved using distilled, de-

[1] U.S. Biomaterials Corp.
[2] Aldrich Chemical, Inc.

TABLE I: COMPOSITION OF BIOGLASSES

Component (wt%)	45S5	52S
SiO_2	45	52
P_2O_5	6	6
CaO	24.5	21
Na_2O	24.5	21

ionized water in a RO-TAP[3] test sieve. Sequential sieve meshes of 25μm, 15μm and 5μm were employed to guarantee particles of <5μm. The resultant powders were each then air dried at 50°C. The HA powder was examined by x-ray analysis using an X-ray Diffractometer[4] which detected no alterations in the sieved HA crystal structure when compared to the as-received HA powder.

Bone stock came from the femur of a game deer harvested within 2 hours of death and stored at 6°C for 24 hours then frozen at –18°C for 48 hours prior to use. The frozen femoral shaft was then sectioned into 11, 1-cm transverse discs, and the soft tissue removed. Processing time was minimized to maintain the bone in a frozen state. The bone discs were wet ground from the sub-periosteal surface to the mid cortex in physiologic, 0.154M NaCl, saline solution using a silicon carbide conical grinding bit at approximately 6,000 rpm with mild hand pressure. The resulting bone particles were next ball milled for 12 hours under refrigerated (3°C) conditions.

The particle sizes for the HA materials and the bone were measured using a laser scattering particle size distribution analyzer[5,6]. The particle radius data for all the synthetic materials and the bone are listed in Table II.

Table II: Particle Radius data for Bioglass, HA and bone in 0.154M saline.

Sample	Mean (μm)	Median (μm)
45S5	1.86	2.64
52S	2.6	4.76
HA	1.46	0.96
bone	0.41	0.31

Methods

To simulate *in vivo* ionic activity between the synthetic materials and bone, both the synthetic materials and bone powders were suspended in 0.2 $^{v}/_{o}$

[3] Tyler RX-29
[4] Scintag 2000
[5] Horiba model LA-910, available at Flint Ink, of Ann Arbor, MI.
[6] Malvern Master Sizer X, Malvern Instruments Ltd.

0.154 M NaCl solution and dispersed using an ultrasonic probe[7] at 70W for 2 minutes. The suitability of *in vitro* studies was addressed by Bagambisa et al.[9] who found that an aqueous *in vitro* model yielded complementary results when compared to the *in vivo* because of the ubiquitous presence of water. ζ-potential measurements for the synthetic materials and bone were made using electrokinetic sonic amplitude (ESA)[8] techniques and collected as a function of pH. The pH was controlled by automatic burette titration of 1M NaOH or 1M HCl into the continuously stirred particle suspension. The particle parameters used during testing are listed in Table III. The viscosity and dielectric constants for the saline solution were estimated to be that of water, 8.92×10^{-4} Pascal-sec and 78.45, respectively, as there are only negligible differences between the viscosity and dielectric constant for water and low concentrations of NaCl solutions[25].

Table III: Bone and HA input data used for ζ-potential determination.

Sample	Density (g/cc)	Particle Radius (μm)
45S5	2.65	1.86
52S	2.65	2.8
HA	3.1	1.46
Bone	2.0	0.41

ζ-potential values at each pH along with the particle size were then used to calculate the stability ratios for homo- and heterocoagulation[26]. The calculations are based on a constant particle charge assumption, and require the input of the dielectric constants for each medium. These constants are listed in Table IV.

Table IV: Dielectric constant values [27-29] and the calculated Hamaker constants.

Sample	Dielectric Constant	Hamaker Constant (J)
45S5	6.9	6.5×10^{-19}
52S	6.9	6.5×10^{-19}
HA	4	1.5×10^{-19}
Bone	17	3.6×10^{-19}
Saline	78.36	4.5×10^{-19}

RESULTS

Zeta Potential

The ζ-potential data as a function of pH for the synthetic materials and bone powders in physiologic saline are shown in Figure 1. The ζ-potential for the 45S5 Bioglass varies from 180 (pH 5) to 25 mV (pH 9) while the 52S Bioglass

[7] Branson Sonifier 250
[8] Matec ESA-8000

maintains a relatively constant potential of ~50 mV in this same pH range. The ζ-potential calculations for the HA powder in physiologic saline showed positive values ranging from 115 to 130mV. The dome-shaped curve, having a maximum ζ-potential at pH 7.0, is similar to the results of Decheyne et al.[30] except that the magnitude of the ζ-potential versus pH data for the current study are uniformly greater. Decheyne et al. report electrophoretic measurements as positive, varying from 0 to 10mV[30]. This variation is attributed to differences in particle size. The current study used crystalline, stoichiometric sieved powders having a mean diameter of 2.91μm while Decheyne et al.[30] used <5μm crystalline, stoichiometric HA powders. Although these particle size differences may appear minor, as previously noted, the magnitude of the ζ-potential is indirectly proportional to the particle diameter through the inertial correction factor $G(\alpha)^{-1}$ as shown in Equation 3. The somewhat larger particle sizes used by Decheyne et al.[30] would yield ζ-potentials that are smaller in magnitude.

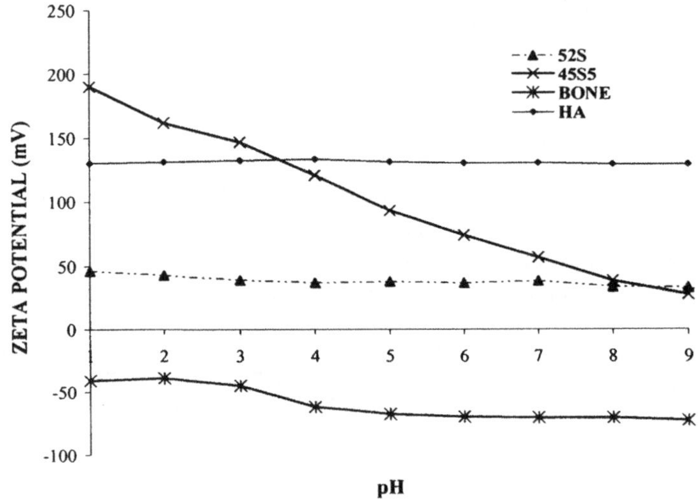

Figure 1: Zeta Potential verses pH for Bone, HA, 45S5 bioglass, and 52S Bioglass from electroacoustic measurements with an electrolyte concentration of 0.154M NaCl and solids content of $0.002^{v}/_{o}$, respectively.

The ζ-potential of the bone varies from –40 to –48 mV throughout the pH range tested. Kowalchuk et al.[25] and Guzelsu et al.[31] studied the ζ-potential of bovine bone using electrophoretic measurements and reported negative values with magnitudes ranging between 0 and 15mV. The lesser ζ-potential value is attributed to differences in particle size and size distribution, bone species, and measurement technique. Kowalchuk et al.[25] reported bone particle diameters as

<5μm, while Guzelsu et al.[31] report particle diameters <10μm. The magnitude of the ζ-potential is indirectly proportional to the particle diameter as discussed earlier. Therefore the larger particle sizes of the powders used by Kowalchuk et al.[25] and Guzelsu et al.[31] account for the lower ζ-potential measurements. Finally, differences in the ζ-potential values may be attributed to differences between bovine and the deer bone used in this study.

Stability Predictions

The stability factor, W, was next calculated for the composite systems (45S5/bone, 52S/bone, HA/bone) using ζ-potential data and plotted as log (W) verses pH in Figures 2-4, respectively. Using a potential barrier of >20 kT to indicate stability, a stability ratio of log (W)>~10 indicates a system which is stable with respect to agglomeration[24]. The stability of the 45S5 Bioglass/bone system is shown in Figure 2 which illustrates that while the individual components (Bioglass and bone) are predicted to remain unagglomerated, the

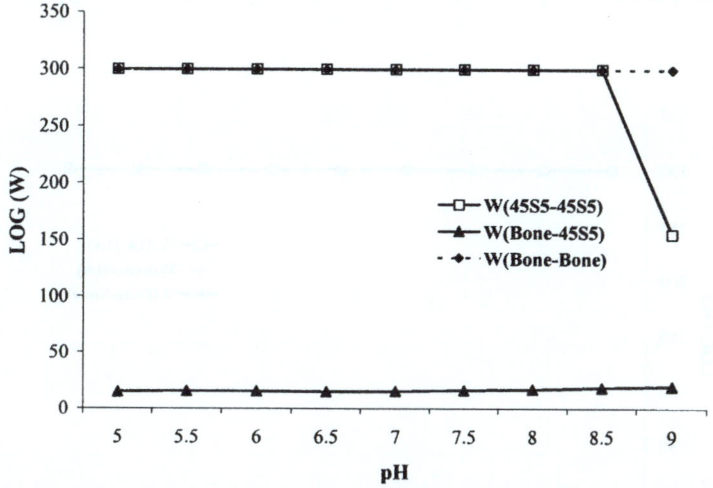

Figure 2: Stability ratio versus pH for bone/45S5 Bioglass using acoustophoretic ζ-potential data at T=30°C.

combination of bone and 45S5 Bioglass are predicted to agglomerate over the pH range tested. In contrast, the higher SiO_2 content 52S Bioglass/bone system shown in Figure 3 shows stability of the individual components and predicts no heteroagglomeration between the components. This agrees with clinical findings that link lower Ca to P molar ratios to a decrease in Bioglass/bone bonding[32]. The

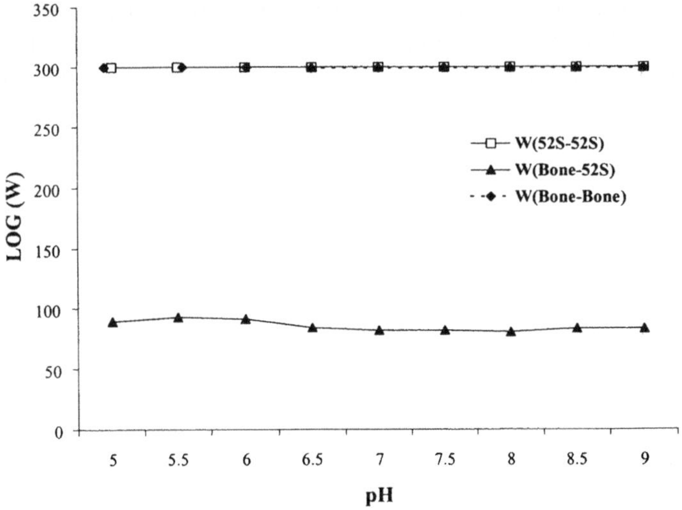

Figure 3: Stability ratio versus pH for bone/52S Bioglass using acoustophoretic ζ-potential data at T=30°C.

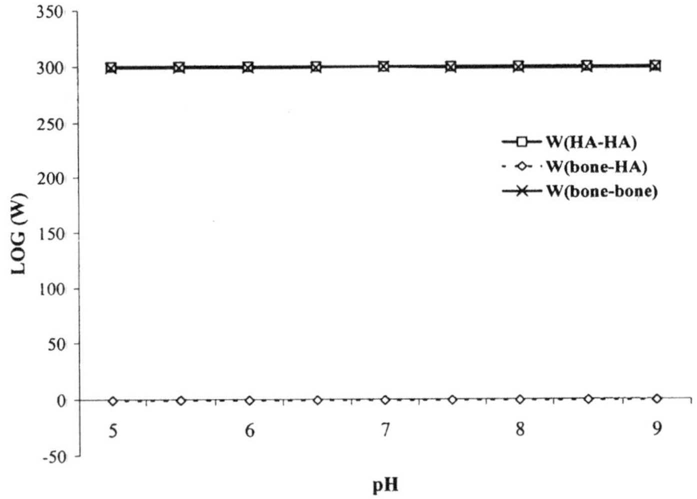

Figure 4: Stability ratio versus pH for bone/HA using acoustophoretic ζ-potential data at T=30°C.

HA/bone system shown in Figure 4 illustrates that both the HA and the bone are stable/unagglomerated with respect to themselves throughout the pH range (5 to

10). However, the composite heterostability shows low, negative values over the pH range investigated. This negative log W value does not correspond to negative stability. Zero stability is the lowest possible stability state. Negative values are an artifact of taking the log of a small stability value. Therefore, from these results, it is expected that HA will agglomerate to bone from pH 5-10.

DISCUSSION

As discussed in an earlier paper[33], the instability of the HA/bone interaction coincides with the mechanisms for physicochemical HA/bone bonding, presented by Bagambisa et al.[9]. Here, the structure of both HA and canine bone are directed by the same calcium and phosphate ionic species present in the calcium phosphate rich layer at the implant surface. Thus, the HA/bone bond must involve strong ionic bonding between these two species. In TEM studies by Bagambisa et al.[9], crystallites of bone were observed to directly bond to the HA surface. Direct HA to bone bonding agrees with the findings of this study which delineated the strong, unstable interaction between HA and bone, resulting in coagulation between these two materials. The heterocoagulation represents a stable interaction whereby the bone-HA interface lies at a thermodynamically lower energy state. The presence of such a stable bonding state predicts a strong mechanical bond since the inherent strength of any material is dependent upon the type and strength of its bonds.

This heterocoagulation behavior over the entire pH range is also significant when the *in vivo* behavior of this system is considered. Normal blood pH is approximately 7.4. In the immediate area around a wound, the pH may be significantly less, creating an acidic environment.

In comparing the ζ-potential versus pH measurements from Decheyne et al.[30] (HA), Kowalchuk et al.[25] (bone) and Guzelsu et al.[31] (bone), the similar appearance of the curves is noted. While differences in the magnitude and sign of the ζ-potential of bone and HA are found to be a function of the particle size, stability calculations invariably indicate an unchanging, unstable interaction between bone and HA at all pHs. This differs from the experimental results of Bagambisa et al.[9] that correlates the bonding zone thickness between bone and HA with changes in pH. For example, at pH 5.19, the HA-bone interaction layer increased but was subsequently resorbed as the pH returned to normal levels. This suggests that while ionic activity may dominate the HA-bone interaction, the cellular *in vivo* environment also plays a role in determining the extent of the initial HA-bone interaction layer.

CONCLUSIONS

Acoustophoretic particle potentials for bone and the synthetic implant materials 45S5 and 52S Bioglass, were measured as a function of pH and converted to ζ-potentials. The stability between 45S5 Bioglass and bone was determined to be unstable, indicating that 45S5 will bond to bone, a finding confirmed by clinical research results. The stability between 52S Bioglass and bone was found to be stable, indicating that 52S will not bond to bone. This has been validated by clinical research citing the decreased interfacial strength between 52S and bone. The differences in bond strength between these 2 Bioglass compositions has been correlated to differing Ca:P ratios leading to changes in their surface potentials that in turn alters the degree of interfacial attraction. While the ζ-potentials for the HA were greater than bone at all pHs tested, both materials are characterized by relatively large ζ-potential values. The strong interaction between HA and bone is predicted for normal blood pH levels and for significant pH deviations and is further evidence to support the presence of a physicochemical bond between HA and bone. These findings agree with those of Bagambisa et al.[9], where crystallites of canine bone were found to be attracted to, and directly bond to HA surfaces. The results of this study reinforce the choice of 45S5 and HA as bioactive materials suitable for use as a bone substitute or as a coating for orthopedic implants[34-37]. Further studies on additional Bioglass compositions along with common orthopedic metals are ongoing.

ACKNOWLEDGEMENTS

The authors would like to acknowledge Daniel Hyduke for his aid in collecting the particle size measurements.

REFERENCES:

1. J. Wilson, A.E. Clark, E. Douek, J. Krieger, W.K. Smith and J. S. Zamet; "Clinical Applications of Bioglass Implants"; P.415 Bioceramics 7. Ed. P.H. Andersson, R.P. Happonen, A.Y. Urpo; Butterworth–Heinemann; Oxford, UK 1994.
2. G.A. Shapoff, D.C. Alexander and A.E. Clark; "Clinical Use of Bioactive Glass Particulate in the Treatment of Human Osseous Defects"; Compound Contin. Educ. Dent., 18[4] 352-63 (1997).
3. J.K. Lobel, "Ossicular Replacement Prosthesis", p.214-36; Clinical Performance of Skeletal Prostheses, Ed. by L.L. Hench and J. Wilson; Chapman and Hall, London, U.K 1996.
4. H.R. Stanley, A.E. Clark, "Using 45S5 Bioglass Cones as Endosseous Ridge Maintenance Implants to Prevent Alveolar Ridge Resorptions – A 5 Year Evaluation", Int. J. of Maxillofac. Implants, 12, 95-105 (1997) .
5. L.L. Hench and J.K. West, "Biological Applications of Bioactive Glasses"., Life Chem. Rep., 13, 187-241 (1996).

6. L.L. Hench and H.A. Pascall, "Histochemical Response at a Biomaterials Interface," *J. Biomed. Mater. Res. Sym.*, **5**, 49-64 (1974).
7. M.Ogiso, H. Kaneda, J. Arasaki and T. Tabata, "Epithelial Attachment and Bone Tissue Formation on the Surface of Hydroxyapatite Dental Implants," in: *Advancements in Biomaterials: Vol 3.*, Chichester: John Wiley and Sons; 1982: 59-64.
8. F.B. Bagambisa, U. Joos and W. Schilli, "The Interaction of Osteogenic Cells with Hydroxyapatite Implant Materials *In Vitro* and *In Vivo*," *Int. J. Oral Maxillofac. Implants*, **5**, 217-226 (1990).
9. F.B. Bagambisa, U. Joos and W. Schilli, "Mechanisms and Structure of the Bond between bone and Hydroxyapatite,' *J. Biomed. Mater. Res.*, **27**, 1047-1055 (1993).
10. J.F. Key, R.H. Doremus and M. Jarcho, "Ion Micromilling of Bone-Implant Interfaces," *Trans. 4th Ann. Meet. Soc. Biomaterials: 10th Int. Biomaterials Symposium*, 154-155 (1978).
11. P.N. DeAza, Z.B. Luklinska, M. Anseau, F. Guitian and S. DeAza, "Morphological Studies of Pseudowollastonite for Biomedical Application," *J. Microsc.*, **182**(4), 24-31 (1996).
12. L.L. Hench, "Bioactive Ceramics"; pp. 54 in Bioceramics: Materials Characteristics Versus *In Vivo* Behavior, Vol. 523. Edited by P. Ducheyne and J. Lemons. Annals N.Y. Acad. Sci. 1988.
13. R.W. O'Brien, "Electro-acoustic Effects in a Dilute Suspension of Spherical Particles," *J. Fluid Mech.*, **190**, 71-86 (1986).
14. R.W. O'Brien, "The Electro-acoustic Equation for a Colloidal Suspension", *J. Fluid Mech.*, **212**,81-93 (1990).
15. T. Oja, Matec Applied Sciences Inc., New York. Personal communication.
16. F.F. Lange, "Powder Processing Science and Technology for Increased Reliability," *J. Am. Ceram. Soc.*, **72**, 3-15 (1989).
17. B.V. Velamekanni and F.F. Lange, "Effect of Interparticle Potentials and Sedimentation on Particle Packing Density of Bimodal Particle Distributions During Pressure Filtration," *J. Am. Ceram. Soc.*, **74**, 166-172, (1991).
18. J.C. Chang, B.V. Velamekanni, F.F. Lange, D.S. Pearson, "Centrafugal Consolidation of Al_2O_3 and Al_2O_3/ZrO_2 Composite Slurries vs. Interparticle Potentials: Particle Packing and Mass Segregation," *J. Am. Ceram. Soc.*, **74**, 2201-2204 (1991).
19. M.J. Crimp and D.A. Oppermann, "Green Density Variations in Relation to Colloidal Packing in SiC/Si_3N_4 Composites," *Proc. Am. Ceram. Soc.: Science, technology, and Applications of Colloidal Suspensions*, 91-101 (1995).
20. M.J. Crimp, "A Novel Approach to Intermetallic Matrix Composite (IMC) Processing," *J. Mater. Sci. Eng.*, **A192/193**, 633-639 (1995).

21. B.V. Derjaguin, L.D. Landau, "Theory of the Stability of Strongly Charged Lyophobic Sols and the Adhesion of Strongly Charged Particles in Solutions of Electrolytes," *Acta Physicochim. URSS.*, **14**, 633 (1941).
22. E.J.W. Verwey and J. Th. G. Overbeek, "Theory of the Stability of the Lyophobic Colloids," Elsevier, Amsterdam, (1948).
23. R. Hogg, T.W. Healy and D.W. Fuerstenau, "Mutual Coagulation of Colloidal Dispersions," *Trans. Faraday Soc.*, **66**, 490 (1966).
24. R.J. Hunter, "Foundations of Colloid Science: Volume 1," Claredon Press, Oxford, 1991.
25. R.M. Kowalchuk, S.R. Pollack and T.A. Corcoran, "Zeta Potential of Bone from Particle Electrophoresis: Solution Composition and Kinetic Effects," *J. Biomed. Mater. Res.*, **29**, 47-57 (1995).
26. B.A. Wilson and M.J. Crimp, "Prediction of Composite Colloidal Suspension Stability Based Upon the Hogg, Healy, and Fuerstenau Interpretation,' *Langmuir*, **9**, 2836-2843 (1993).
27. J.B. Park and R.S. Lakes, "Biomaterials: An Introduction, 2nd Edition," Plenum Press, New York, 1992, 122-125, 317-352.
28. S. Hontsu, T.Matsumoto, J.Ishii, M. Nakamori, H. Tabata and T. Kawai, "Electrical Properties of Hydroxyapitite Thin Films Grown by Pulsed Laser Deposition," *J. Thin Solid Films*, **295**, 214-217 (1997).
29. H. Maeda, "Effect of Water on Piezoelectric, Dielectric, and Elastic Properties of Bone," *Biopolymers*, **21**, 2055-2068 (1982).
30. R. Ducheyne, C.S. Kim and S.R. Pollack, " The Effect of Phase Differences on the Time Dependent Variation of the Zeta Potential of Hydroxyapatite," *J. Biomed. Mater. Res.*, **26**, 147-168 (1992).
31. N. Guzelsu and R.L. Regimbal, "The Origin of Electrokinetic Potentials in Bone Tissue: The Organic Phase," *J. Biomech.*, **23**(7), 661-672 (1990).
32. L.L. Hench and H.A. Paschall, "Direct Chemical Bonding Between Bio-active Glass-Ceramic Materials and Bone", *J. Biomed. Maters. Res. Symp.*, **4**, 25-42 (1973).
33. D.A. Oppermann, M.J. Crimp and D.M. Bement, "*In vitro* Stability Predictions for the Bone/Hydroxyapatite Composite System", *J. Biomed. Mater. Res.*, **42**, [3], 412-416 (1998).
34. Y. Kakutani, T. Yamamuro and T. Nakamura, "Strengthening of Bone-Implant Interface by the use of Granule Coatings on Alumina Ceramics," *J. Biomed. Mater. Res.*, **23**, 781-808 (1989).
35. H. Oonishi, M. Yamamuro, H. Ishimaru, E. Tsuji, S. Kushitani, M. Aono and Y. Ukon, "The Effect of Hydroxyapatite Coating on Bone Growth into Porous Titanium Alloy Implants," *J. Bone Joint Surg.*, **71-B**(2), 213-216 (1989).

36. M. Jarcho, J.F. Kay, K.T. Gumaer, R.H. Doremus and H.P. Drobeck, "Tissue, Cellular and Sub-cellular Events at a Bone-Ceramic Hydroxyapatite Interface," *J.Bioeng.*, **1**, 79-92 (1976).
37. L.L. Hench, R.J. Splinter, W.C. Allen and T.K. Greenlee, "Bonding Mechanism at the Interface of Ceramic Prosthetic Materials," *J. Biomed. Mater. Res.*, **2**(1), 117-141 (1972).

GLASS-HYDROXYAPATITE COATINGS ON TITANIUM-BASED IMPLANTS

J.M. Gomez-Vega, E. Saiz and A.P. Tomsia
Materials Sciences Division, Lawrence Berkeley National Laboratory, Berkeley MS 62-203, CA 94720, USA

G.W. Marshall and S.J. Marshall
Department of Restorative Dentistry, University of California, San Francisco 707 Parnassus Ave, D-2246, CA 94143, USA

ABSTRACT

Glasses in the system Si-Ca-Na-Mg-P-K-O that match the thermal expansion coefficient of Ti6Al4V were prepared by optimizing their composition. The synthesized glasses were used to coat the titanium alloy by an enameling technique.

Glass-hydroxyapatite (HA) coatings were fabricated in two different ways: embedding HA particles on the surface of the coatings, and firing mixtures of glass powder and HA particles. The fabricated coatings showed excellent adhesion to the substrate and they were able to form apatite on their surfaces when tested *in vitro* by soaking in a simulated body fluid (SBF).

INTRODUCTION

Ti6Al4V is one of the most widely used alloys for the fabrication of implants where body loads are important, such as hip prosthesis.[1] Nonetheless, Ti6Al4V is a bioinert material whose adherence to the bone is very low, so the use of coatings has been considered as a manner to improve their adhesion.[2] Plasma spraying of HA is the most used and studied method, but it fails to produce reliable and long lasting coatings due to weak metal/HA interfaces.[3,4]

Previous works have indicated that silicate-based glasses can be successfully used to coat Ti6Al4V by an enameling technique.[5,6] However, when tested *in vitro*, the capability of these glasses to form apatite on their surfaces is very limited due to their high silica content (≥ 57 wt%). Therefore, this work explores the use of glass-HA composite coatings in order to improve their bioactivity, while at the same time maintaining good adhesion to the metal.

EXPERIMENTAL

Glasses were prepared by mixing and firing the required oxides using a standard procedure.[7] The composition and main thermal properties of the glasses used in this work and HA are listed in Table I.

Table I. Composition and main properties of the synthesized glasses and HA

	Composition (wt%)						α	Ts
	SiO_2	Na_2O	CaO	MgO	P_2O_5	K_2O	(10^{-6} °C^{-1})	(°C)
6P55	54.5	12.0	15.0	8.5	6.0	4.0	11.0	602
6P57	56.5	11.0	15.0	8.5	6.0	3.0	10.8	609
6P61	61.1	10.3	12.6	7.2	6.0	2.8	10.2	624
6P68	67.7	8.3	10.1	5.7	6.0	2.2	8.8	644
HA*							~14.0	

α = Coefficient of thermal expansion (measured between 200 and 400°C).
$\alpha_{Ti6Al4V} \approx 9.6 \cdot 10^{-6}$ °C^{-1}
Ts = Softening point.
*HA = $Ca_{10}(PO_4)_6(OH)_2$ is a double salt of tricalcium phosphate and calcium hydroxide.

Ti6Al4V (99% purity, President Titanium, Hanson MA) plates (15×10×1 mm) were ground with silicon carbide paper (600 grit) and cleaned with acetone and ethanol prior to their use. To manufacture the coatings, a glass powder (particle diameter <30 μm) suspension in ethanol was poured onto the plates placed in a beaker, and allowed to settle completely for several hours. HA (99% purity, Fluka) particles were added in two ways (i) a suspension of HA particles (diameter 50-150 μm) in ethanol was gently poured to cover approximately 15-20% of the coating surface, and (ii) a suspension in ethanol of a mixture (50:50 wt%) of glass-HA particles (diameter <30 μm) was deposited as a second layer. Coatings with two glass-HA composite layers one on top of the other were also fabricated, with 20 and 40 wt% of HA, respectively. Once the sedimentation concluded, the liquid was carefully extracted with a pipette, and the beaker was placed in an oven at 75°C overnight to dry the green-coatings completely. The green-coatings prepared as indicated were fired in air in a Unitek dental furnace according to the optimum conditions established in previous work:[6] furnace preheating to 600°C, temperature ramp 40°C/min in low vacuum (~10^{-3} Pa), to the final temperature 800-840°C, dwell time 30 s, and quenching.

The strength of the glass/metal and glass/HA interfaces was qualitatively evaluated by Vickers indentations on the coating cross sections with 0.2 Kg load in air. The *in vitro* behavior of the coatings was tested by immersion in a simulated body fluid (SBF) at 37°C for times up to 52 days.[8] The coating surfaces and polished cross sections were examined by scanning electron microscopy with associated wavelength dispersive analysis (SEM-WDS).

RESULTS AND DISCUSSION

The aim of this work was to coat Ti6Al4V with glass-HA composites in order to enhance the adaptation of this metal to the body when used in implants. The coating fulfills two purposes: it prevents the metal from being corroded by the body fluids, and promotes adhesion to the bone (when the coating is bioactive). The presence of HA particles in the glass coatings has been studied as a way to enhance their bioactivity, provided that strong glass/metal interfaces were maintained.

It was possible to fabricate coatings with thicknesses ranging from 50 to 150 μm with glasses 6P68, 6P61 and 6P57 since the thermal stress induced by the difference in α with Ti6Al4V was not enough to crack the coatings.[6]

The first approach to the incorporation of HA particles into the coatings consisted of HA particle deposition on top of the glass, which exhibits good adhesion to the metal. More details about processing can be found elsewhere.[9] For example, the surface of glass 6P68 coating with HA particles embedded is shown in Figure 1. HA particles do not melt at the firing temperature used, so they only immerse partially into the glass when it softens, keeping their shape and remaining attached to the glass coating after cooling. Vickers indentations on the cross sections of 6P57 coating with embedded HA particles indicate that both glass/Ti6Al4V and glass/HA interfaces are strong as the cracks never propagate along the interfaces but tend to be driven into the glass or across the particles (Figure 2). The maximum concentration of particles which can be embedded in the coating is controlled by the induced stress since HA has a higher α value than the glasses (Table I). Coverage of coating surface <20% and interparticle distances higher than the particle diameter resulted in crack-free coatings.[9]

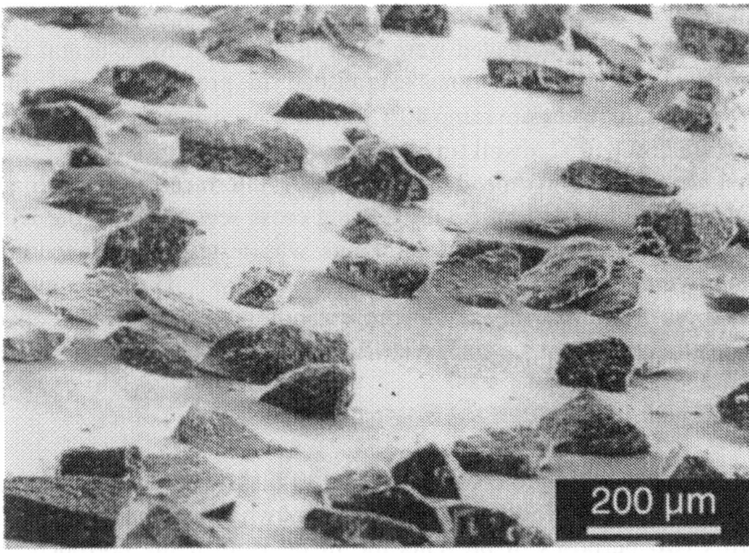

Figure 1. Surface of glass 6P68 coating with embedded HA particles.

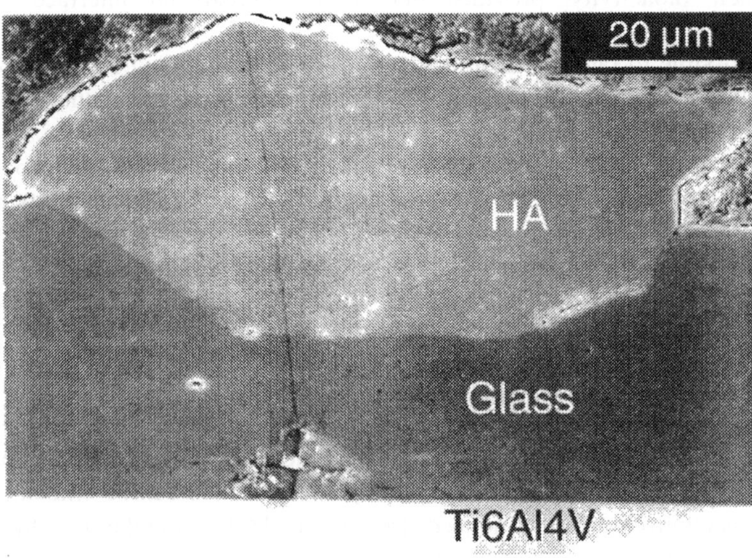

Figure 2. Vickers indentation on cross sections of 6P57 coating with embedded HA particles.

The second method used to incorporate HA in the coatings was to deposit glass-HA composite mixtures as layers on a glass layer that is well-bonded to the metal substrate. This multilayer approach allows fabrication of coatings with a positive and controllable gradient in HA concentration towards the exterior and, therefore, a similar gradient in bioactivity.[10] For example, in the cross section of a three layered coating (with each layer~25 μm thickness) of glass 6P61 with 0, 20 and 40 wt% of HA, respectively, a gradient in HA concentration in the coating can be observed (Figure 3). Some segregation by particle sizes is evident and smaller particles are found mainly in the external part of the coating. Due to the high viscosity of the glass and high density of HA as compared to the glasses, the expected segregation during firing should be in the opposite direction. Therefore, the segregation of small particles took place during the sedimentation process.

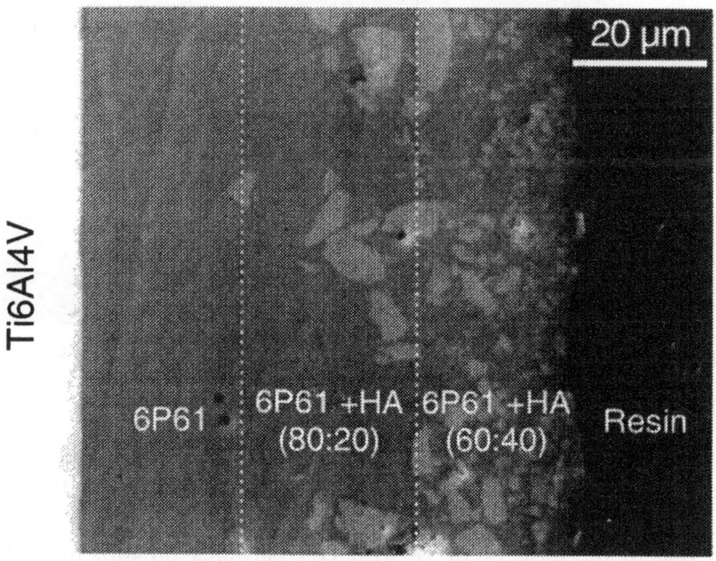

Figure 3. Cross-section of a three-layered coating of glass 6P61 with 0, 20 and 40 wt% HA particles, respectively.

The Si and Ca line profiles along the coating 6P57/(6P57+HA) only shows the sharp transition at the glass/HA interfaces, following their composition (Figure 4). Consequently, there is no reaction or interdiffusion at the glass/HA interface at the temperatures used, in agreement with previous work where no reaction product was found at temperatures < 850°C.[11]

No cracks were detected either at the glass/HA or glass/metal interfaces, so the coatings were able to withstand the tension created by the HA particles. However, some cracks along the coating were originated after cutting the samples to prepare the cross sections, which indicates that the coatings were under high stress. Lower particle concentration and/or size should be also considered to reduce tension in the coating, and a compromise between bioactivity and integrity of the coatings should be established.

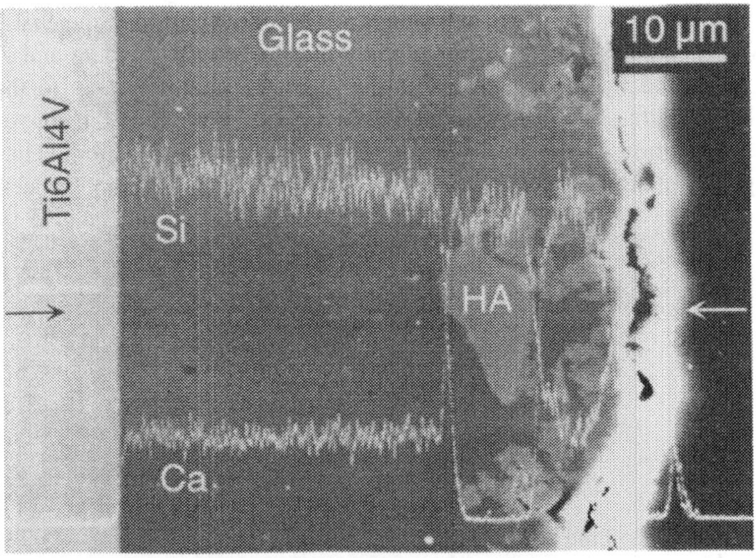

Figure 4. SEM-WDS line analysis (between arrows) of elements Si and Ca along the coating 6P57/(6P57+HA).

When tested *in vitro*, it was observed that an apatite precipitated on the coating surfaces after 30 days in SBF. The precipitation of apatite on composite coatings 6P57/(6P57+HA) was uniform and covered most of its surface (Figure 5). However, in the case of 6P57 with HA particles on top, nucleation of the apatite started on the HA particles, and covered large regions of the glass surface around the particles when the time of immersion was extended over 30 days (Figure 6). It was found that the coating surface was enriched in Ca and P as time of immersion was increased and, once apatite nucleated, it spread readily over the rest of the glass surface.[8] The effect of SBF on a coating where a crack is present, as when two particles are too close, is illustrated in Figure 7. It can be observed that, with a crack present between the two particles, the fluid could corrode the coating and reach the metal. Therefore, the processing conditions of this methodology, especially size, concentration and distribution of particles, must be optimized in order to fabricate crack-free coatings.

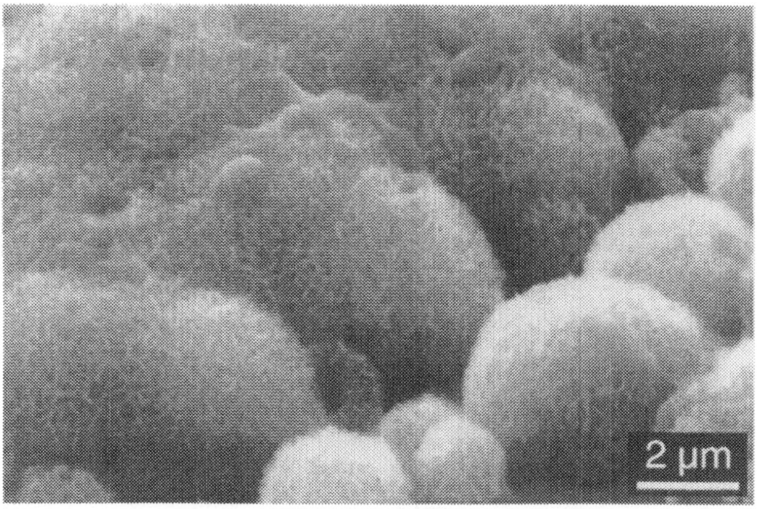

Figure 5. Detail of the formed apatite on 6P57/(6P57+HA) coating after 30 days in SBF.

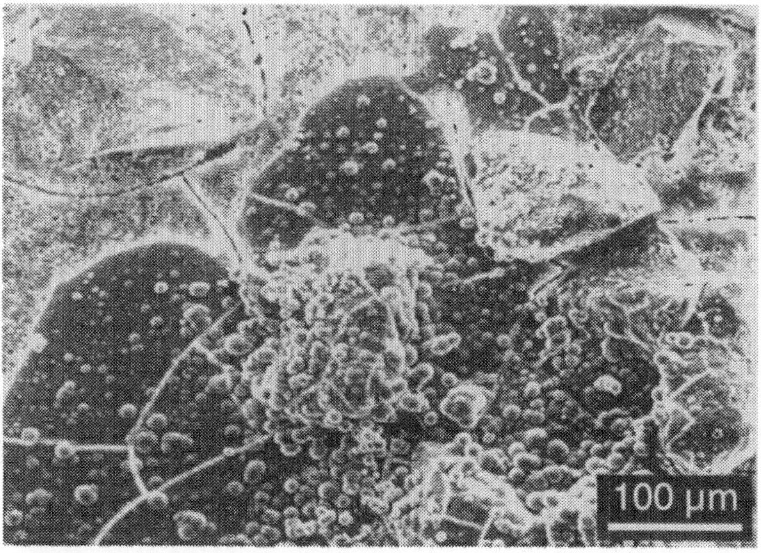

Figure 6. Precipitated apatite on 6P57 glass coating with HA particles after immersion in SBF for 52 days.

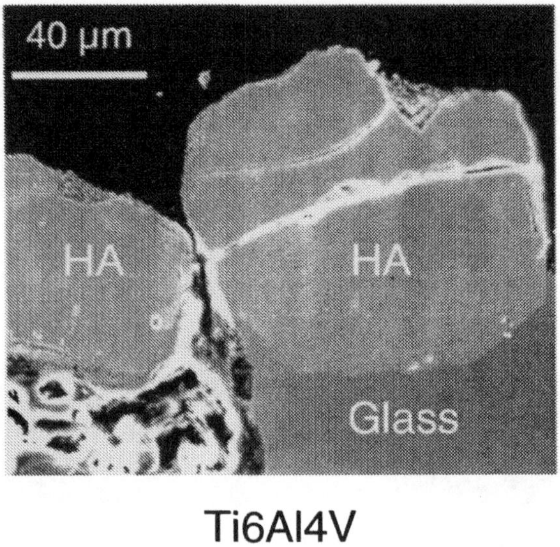

Figure 7. Cross section of coating 6P57 with HA particles embedded on top after immersion in SBF for 15 days.

CONCLUSIONS

Ti6Al4V could be coated with glass-HA composites by an enameling technique. HA was incorporated by deposition of particles, or layers of glass-HA mixtures, on top of a glass layer with strong adhesion to the metal. During *in vitro* tests, apatite formed on their surfaces after 30 days in SBF, which suggests that good osteointegration could be achieved when tested *in vivo*.

The fabrication of glass-HA coatings on Ti6Al4V provides a new approach to stable and long-lasting implants. The glass coating fulfills a double objective since it protects the metal from corrosion and improves the adhesion to the bone. With this methodology, it should be possible to design the coating for each type of implant by optimization of variables such as glass composition, thickness, size, shape and gradient of particle concentration along the coating.

ACKNOWLEDGEMENTS

This work was supported by NIH/NIDR Grant 1R01DE11289. Jose M. Gomez-Vega wishes to thank FICYT for the postdoctoral fellowship given to him in the II Plan Regional de Investigación del Principado de Asturias (Spain).

REFERENCES

[1]L.L. Hench, "Bioceramics: from concept to clinic", *Journal of the American Ceramic* Society, 74 [7] 1487-1510 (1991).

[2]T. Kitsugi, T. Nakamura, M. Oka, Y. Senaha, T. Goto and T. Shibuya, "Bone-bonding behavior of plasma-sprayed coatings of Bioglass®, AW-glass ceramic, and tricalcium phosphate on titanium alloy," *Journal of Biomedical Materials Research*, 30 [2] 261-269 (1996).

[3]W.R. Lacefield, "Hydroxylapatite coating"; pp. 223-238 in *An Introduction to Bioceramics.* Edited by L.J. Hench and J. Wilson, World Scientific, Singapore 1993.

[4]W. Suchanek and M. Yoshimura, "Processing and properties of hydroxyapatite-based biomaterials for use as hard tissue replacement implants," *Journal of Materials Research*, 13 [1] 94-117 (1998).

[5]A. Pazo, E. Saiz and A.P. Tomsia, "Silicate glass coatings on Ti-based implants," *Acta Materialia*, 46 [7] 2551-2558 (1998).

[6]J.M. Gomez-Vega, E. Saiz and A.P. Tomsia, "Bioactive glass-based coatings for titanium implants alloys," *Journal of Biomedical Materials Research* (in press).

[7]A. Pazo, E. Saiz and A.P. Tomsia, "Bioactive coatings on Ti and Ti6Al4V alloys for medical applications"; pp. 543-550 in *Ceramic Microstructures.* Edited by A.P. Tomsia and A.M. Glaeser, Plenum Press, New York, 1998.

[8]J.M. Gomez-Vega, E. Saiz, A.P. Tomsia, G.W. Marshall and S.J. Marshall, "Bioactive glass coatings with hydroxyapatite and Bioglass® particles on Ti-based implants. 2. *In vitro* behavior," *Biomaterials* (submitted).

[9]J.M. Gomez-Vega, E. Saiz, A.P. Tomsia, G.W. Marshall and S.J. Marshall, "Bioactive glass coatings with hydroxyapatite and Bioglass® particles on Ti-based implants. 1. Processing," *Biomaterials* (submitted).

[10]J.M. Gomez-Vega, E. Saiz, A.P. Tomsia, G.W. Marshall and S.J. Marshall, "A multilayer approach to fabricate bioactive glass coatings on Ti alloys," in *Biomedical Materials-Drug Delivery, Implants and Tissue Engineering*. Edited by T. Neenan, M. Marcolongo and R.F. Valentini, *Materials Research Society Proceedings,* Vol. 550, 1999 (in press).

[11]A.P. Tomsia, J.S. Moya and F. Guitian, "New route for hydroxyapatite coatings on Ti-based human implants," *Scripta Metalurgica et Materialia*, 31 [8] 995-1000 (1994).

SYNTHESIS OF HYDROXYAPATITE VIA MECHANICAL ACTIVATION

K.C.B. Yeong[1], J. Wang[1], S.C. Ng[2]
[1]Department of Materials Science, [2]Department of Physics
Faculty of Science, National University of Singapore
Singapore 119260

ABSTRACT

Fine hydroxyapatite (HA) precursor powders were prepared by mechanically activating a powder mixture of calcium oxide (CaO) and brushite ($CaHPO_4.2H_2O$) in a high-energy shaker mill. Highly crystalline hydroxyapatite particles were formed when the activated powder was thermally treated at a temperature as low as 800 °C. A sintered density of 97.50% theoretical and hardness of 5.00 GPa were measured for the hydroxyapatite derived from mechanical activation and sintered at 1200 °C. Similar heat treatment of the starting powder composition that was not subjected to any mechanical activation did not result in the formation of a crystalline hydroxyapatite.

INTRODUCTION

Hydroxyapatite [$Ca_{10}(PO_4)_6(OH)_2$, HA] is the main mineral constituent of vertebrate skeletal systems [1]. As a bioceramic material, it has been employed in many biomedical applications, such as implants and coatings onto prosthesis, due to its excellent biocompatibility and bioactivity [2-4]. Sintered hydroxyapatite can be fabricated via a number of ceramic processing routes [5-10], although the resulting microstructure and properties vary considerably from one route to another. In search for a reliable processing technique to prepare a fine and sintering-reactive powder for fabrication of sintered hydroxyapatites, a novel mechanical activation route is reported in this paper. In the past, attempts were made to synthesize hydroxyapatite through mechano-chemical reactions [11,12].

However, they resulted in the formation of either a calcium-deficient HA, which upon calcination at ~720 °C for developing a crystalline phase led to the occurrence of β-tricalcium phosphate (β-TCP) [11], or a mixture consisting of HA and β-TCP [12]. The objectives of this work are twofold: (a) to synthesize a highly crystalline HA by calcining a mechanically activated powder mixture consisting of CaO and $CaHPO_4.2H_2O$; and (b) to investigate the effects of processing parameters involved, such as the activation time, calcination and sintering temperatures, on the sintered density, microstructure and mechanical properties of the activation-derived hydroxyapatite.

EXPERIMENTAL PROCEDURES

The starting materials for mechanical activation were commercially available brushite ($CaHPO_4.2H_2O$, Merck) and calcium oxide (CaO, G.C.E.). Appropriate amounts of these starting materials for a molar ratio of 3:2 were loaded into an alumina vial of 37 mm in diameter and 40 mm in length together with a stainless steel ball of 12.7 mm in diameter and the mechanical activation was carried out in a shaker mill for various time periods. Phases present in the powder compositions activated for various time periods were analyzed using an X-ray diffractometer (CuKα, X'pert Diffractometer, Philips). Their particle sizes were estimated on the basis of specific surface areas, as measured using a BET surface area analyzer (NOVA 2000, Quantachrome). Thermal analyses (TGA, DTA) of the mechanically-activated powders were carried out at a heating rate of 10 °C/minute in air from room temperature to 900 °C (Dupont 2100 thermal analyze). Particle morphologies were studied using a transmission electron microscope (JOEL, 100CX). To fabricate sintered hydroxyapatites, the powder mechanically-activated for 30 hours was de-agglomerated in a conventional ball mill for 24 hours in ethanol in order to remove hard agglomerates. The powder was then uniaxially pressed into pellets in a hardened steel die of 10 mm in diameter at a pressure of 25 MPa, followed by isostatic pressing at a pressure of 345 MPa, prior to being sintered at various temperatures in the range of 900 to 1300 °C. Both heating and cooling rates were fixed at 5 °C/minute. The sintered hydroxyapatite pellets were then characterized for density using the Archimedes method in distilled water, into which a few drops of wetting agent was added. They were then polished to 6 μm finish using diamond paste and tested for Vickers' hardness using indentation technique (Shimadzu HSV-20). Scanning electron microscope (SEM, Philips XL30) was then employed to study both the polished and fracture surfaces of sintered hydroxyapatites.

RESULTS AND DISCUSSION

Figure 1 shows the XRD traces for the powder mixtures of CaO and $CaHPO_4.2H_2O$ subjected to mechanical activation for various time periods ranging from 5 to 30 hours, together with that of the starting powder that was not subjected to any mechanical activation. For the starting powder mixture that was not subjected to any mechanical activation, only sharp peaks of crystalline CaO, $CaHPO_4.2H_2O$ and $CaHPO_4$ are observed in the XRD trace, indicating that little or no reaction occurred during the mixing milling in the conventional ball mill. The occurrence of $CaHPO_4$ in the starting powder mixture is attributed to the dehydration of $CaHPO_4.2H_2O$ when the powder mixture was dried following ball milling for 5 hours. For the powder that was subjected to 5 hours of mechanical activation, in contrast, almost all the sharp peaks that was of CaO, $CaHPO_4.2H_2O$ and $CaHPO_4$ have vanished, and they are replaced by a few broadened ones.

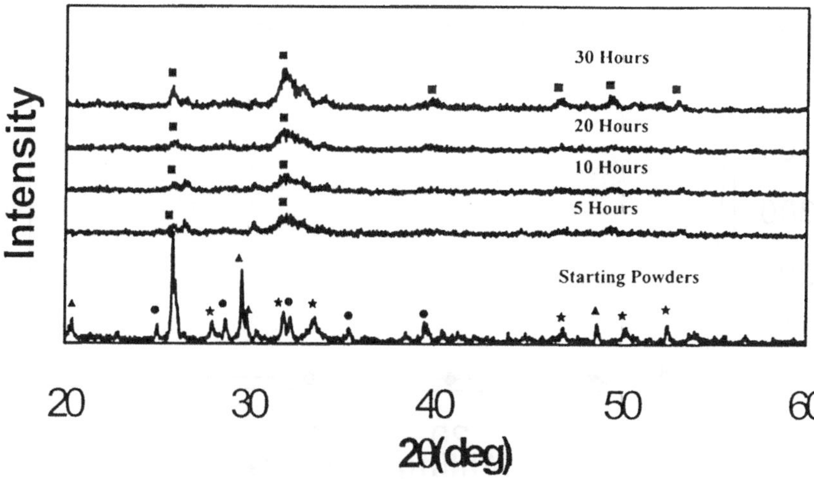

Fig. 1: XRD patterns of the powder mixtures consisting of calcium oxide (CaO) and brushite ($CaHPO_4.2H_2O$) subjected to 0-30 hours of mechanical activation. (▲ : $CaHPO_4.2H_2O$, ● : $CaHPO_4$, ★ : CaO, ■ : HA)

The most prominent one situated at the 2θ angle of ~32° corresponds to hydroxyapatite (211) peak and this indicates that either an amorphous or nanocrystalline hydroxyapatite phase has been formed as a result of mechanical activation. With increasing activation time, up to 30 hours, there is a steady increase in the crystallinity of fine hydroxyapatite crystallites, as evidenced by the increase in (211) peak intensity. The average crystallite size of the powder mechanically activated for 30 hours was estimated to be ~8 nm using the Scherrer formula [13] on the basis of half peak breadth of HA (211). The particle sizes of the powder mixtures that were subjected to various hours of mechanical activation were estimated on the basis of BET surface areas. As shown in Figure 2, a fall in particle size was seen, from ~550 nm for the starting powder mixture to ~40 nm for the powder that was subjected to 2 hours of mechanical activation. Prolonged mechanical activation up to 30 hours resulted in little further refinement in the particle size, although the hydroxyapatite phase was further established with increasing activation time. This suggests that the initial mechanical activation led to fragmentation of the starting powder particles together with a degree of amorphization as indicated by the much-broadened XRD peaks. The formation of nanocrystalline hydroxyapatite was then triggered in a highly activated powder matrix.

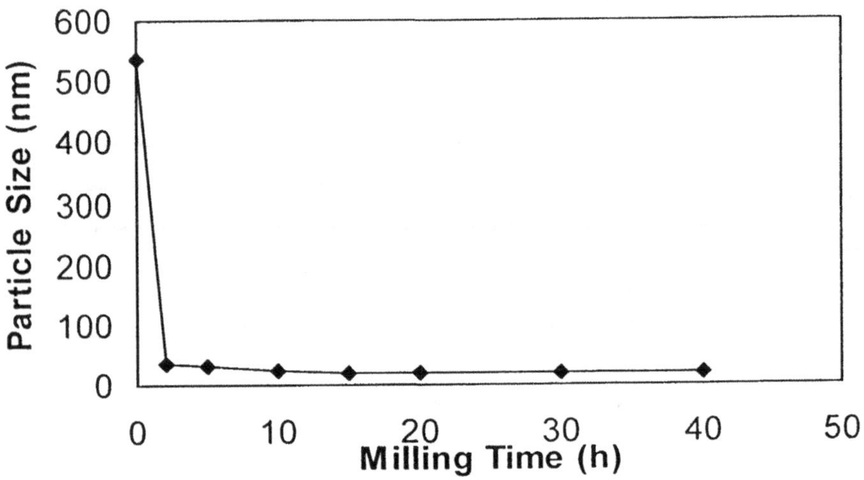

Fig. 2: Particle size as a function of milling time based on estimations obtained from BET results.

Figure 3(a) is a SEM micrograph showing the powder subjected to 30 hours of mechanical activation. It consists of particle agglomerates of varying size in the range of 0.5-1.0 μm. Nanosized spherical particles are clearly visible within each of the agglomerates and this corresponds well with the broadened XRD peaks. In contrast, the powders that were not subjected to any mechanical activation consist of large, irregular agglomerates of CaO together with elongated particles of $CaHPO_4.2H_2O$.

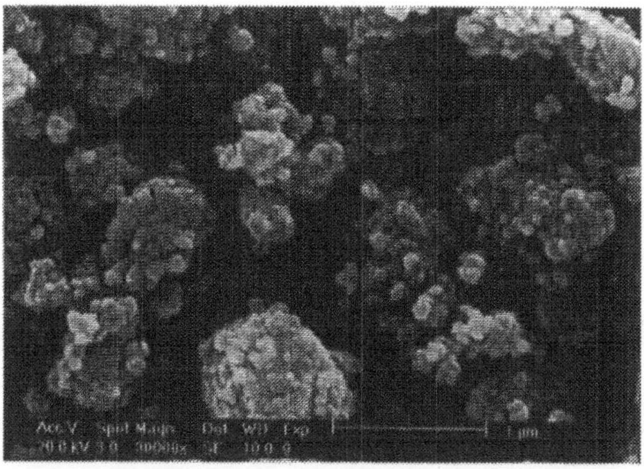

Fig. 3 (a): SEM micrographs of powders after 30 hours of mechanical activation.

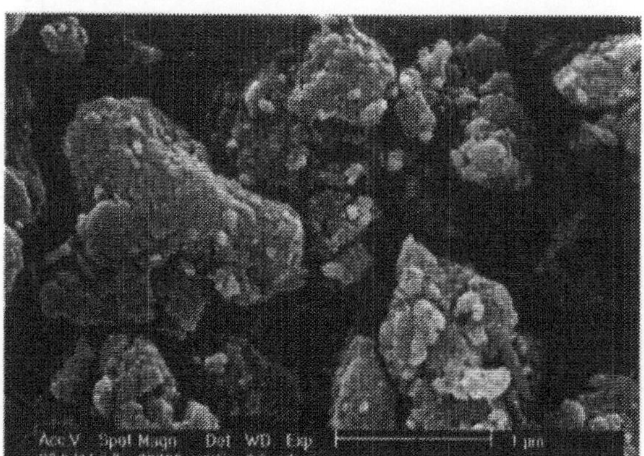

Fig. 3 (b): SEM micrographs of powders not subjected to any mechanical activation.

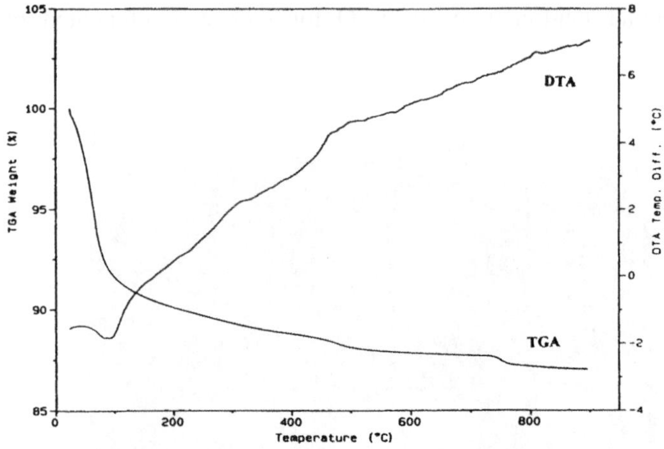

Fig. 4 (a): DTA, TGA trace of powders subjected to 30 hours of mechanical activation.

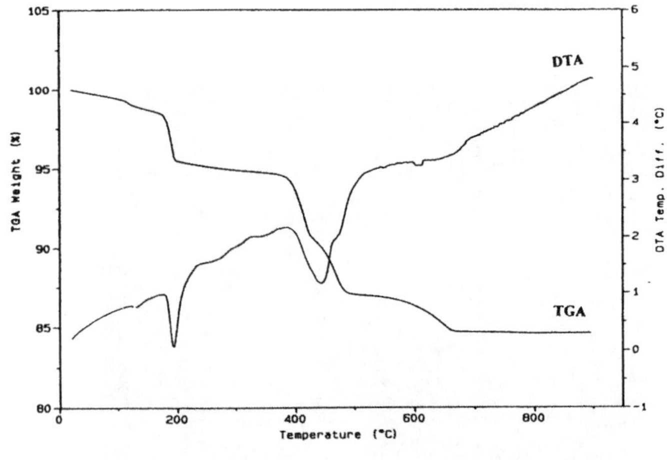

Fig. 4 (b): DTA, TGA trace of powders not subjected to any mechanical activation.

Figure 4(a) shows the TGA and DTA curves at a heating rate of 10 °C/min in air for the powder that was subjected to 30 hours of mechanical activation. The major weight loss occurs at temperatures below 100 °C, due to the elimination of residual water. This corresponds to a broadened endothermic reaction over the same temperature range. In contrast, the powder that was not subjected to any mechanical activation exhibits two endothermic reactions at 194 °C and 444 °C respectively, corresponding to two weight losses over the same temperature ranges. They are due to the loss of water in association with the conversion from $CaHPO_4.2H_2O$ to $CaHPO_4$ and the transformation of $CaHPO_4$ to γ-$Ca_2P_2O_7$, respectively [14]. These thermoanalytical results agree with those obtained previously for the mechanochemically synthesized calcium-deficient apatite [15]. This indicates that 30 hours of mechanical activation has more or less completed the reaction between CaO and $CaHPO_4.2H_2O$, at room temperature. Figure 5(a) is a bright field TEM micrograph showing the starting powder mixture that was not subjected to mechanical activation. It consists of large, elongated particles of $CaHPO_4.2H_2O$ having an average size of ~3 μm together with small irregularly-shaped CaO particles.

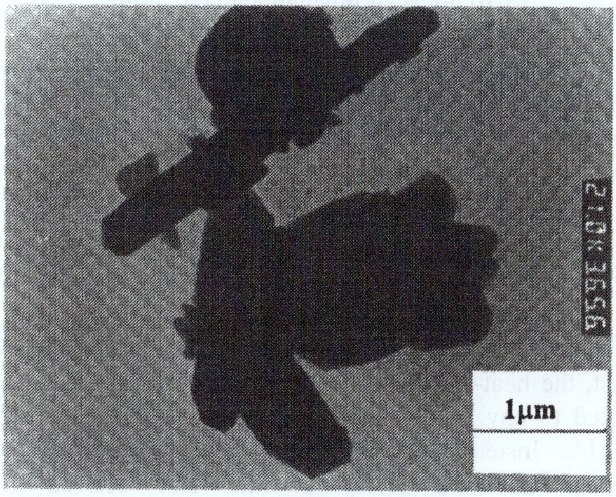

Fig. 5 (a): TEM of starting powders not subjected to any mechanical activation.

As a comparison, Figure 5(b) shows the hydroxyapatite powder synthesized by 30 hours of mechanical activation. It consists of rather well dispersed nanocrystallites of hydroxyapatite, which exhibits an oval shape and a particle size of ~20 nm.

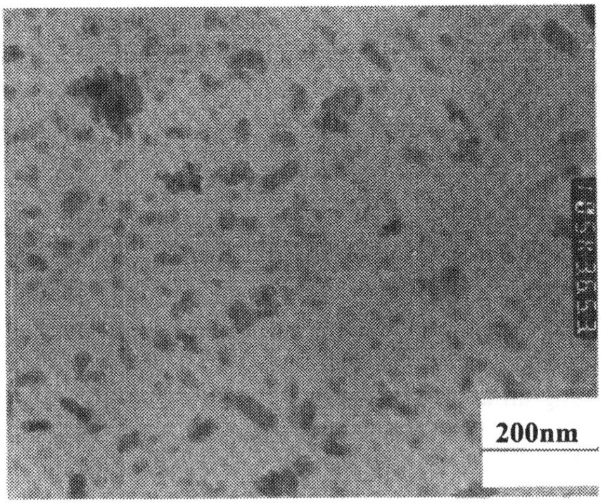

Fig. 5 (b): TEM of starting powders subjected to 30 hours of mechanical activation.

As expected, a thermal treatment at increasing temperature in the range of 400 °C to 800 °C resulted in an increase in crystallinity as shown in Figures 6(a,b,c). However, for the powder that was mechanically activated for a time period of less than 30 hours, HA was hardly formed upon increasing heat treatment. Instead, crystalline β-TCP was developed. This can be attributed to an insufficient activation time resulting in the incomplete reaction of γ-$Ca_2P_2O_7$, which reacts with the hydroxyl ions derived from the dehydroxylation of HA at ~800 °C, to form β-TCP [12]. As can be seen in Figure 6(c), the powder that was mechanically activated for 30 hours was a highly crystalline HA upon calcined at 800 °C for 1 hour. In contrast, the heat-treatment at the same temperature of the powder that was not subjected to any mechanical activation did not result in the complete formation of HA. Instead, it is a mixture consisting of CaO, $CaHPO_4$, $CaHPO_4.2H_2O$, β-TCP and HA. For the HA derived from brushite ($CaHPO_4.2H_2O$) and calcium oxide (CaO), the mechanical activation led to a lower formation temperature, when compared to those previously reported [17].

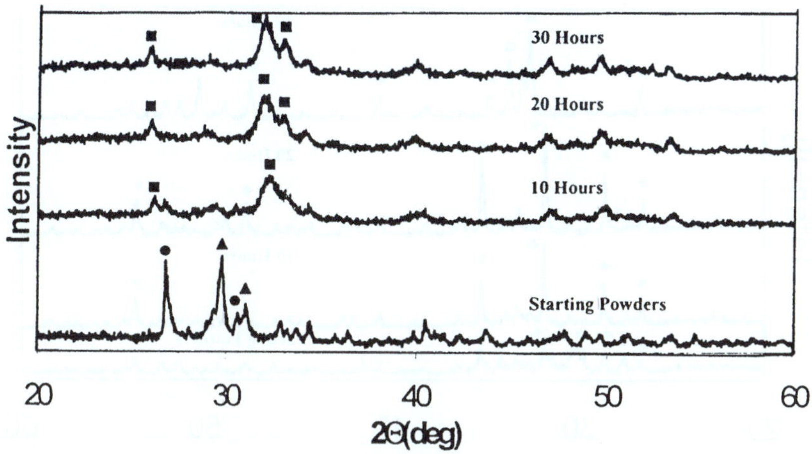

Fig. 6 (a): XRD traces of powders subjected to various time periods of mechanical activation from 0-30 hours and calcined at 400 °C.
(▲ : $CaHPO_4.2H_2O$, ● : $CaHPO_4$, ■ : HA)

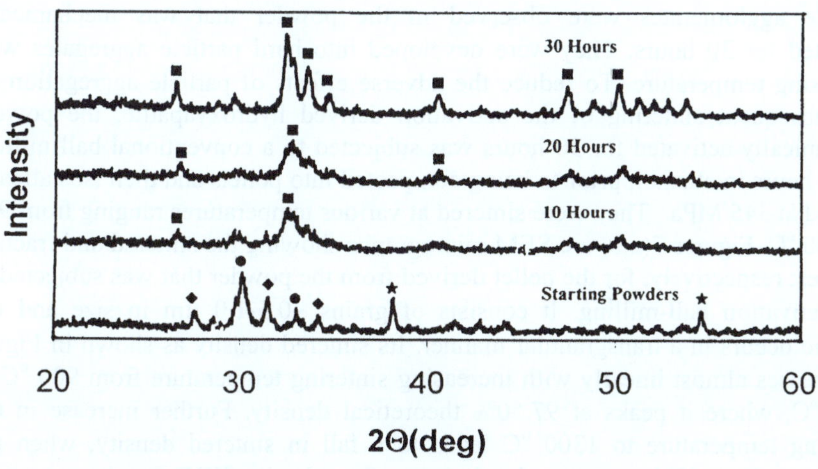

Fig. 6 (b): XRD traces of powders subjected to various time periods of mechanical activation from 0-30 hours and calcined at 600 °C.
(▲ : $CaHPO_4.2H_2O$, ● : $CaHPO_4$, ★ : CaO, ■ : HA, ◆ : β-TCP)

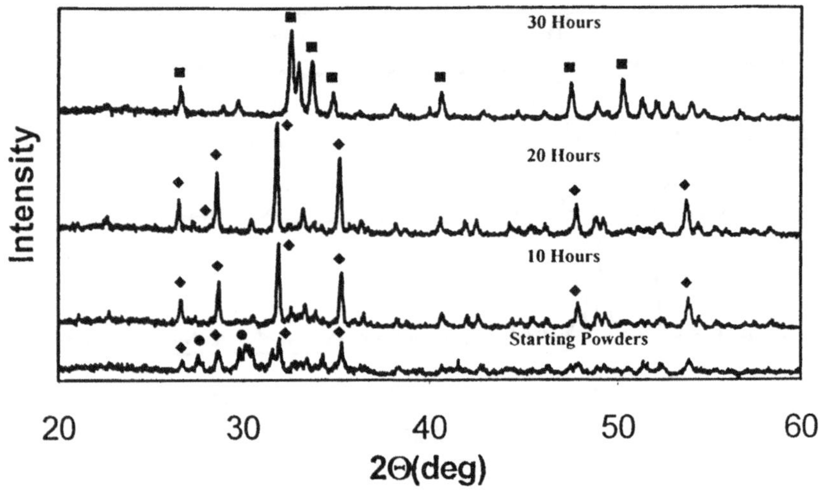

Fig. 6 (c): XRD traces of powders subjected to various time periods of mechanical activation from 0-30 hours and calcined at 800 °C.
(▲ : $CaHPO_4.2H_2O$, ● : $CaHPO_4$, ■ : HA, ◆: β-TCP)

Particle agglomerates were observed in the powder that was mechanically activated for 30 hours. They were developed into hard particle aggregates with increasing temperature. To reduce the adverse effects of particle aggregation on the subsequent sintering of the activation derived hydroxyapatite, the powder mechanically activated for 30 hours was subjected to a conventional ball milling for 24 hours in ethanol, prior to being compacted into pellets and then isostatically pressed at 345 MPa. They were sintered at various temperatures ranging from 900 to 1300 °C. Figures 7(a,b) are SEM micrographs showing the sintered and fracture surfaces; respectively, for the pellet derived from the powder that was subjected to post-activation ball-milling. It consists of grains ~0.5-1.0 μm in size and the fracture occurs in a transgranular manner. Its sintered density as shown in Figure 8, increases almost linearly with increasing sintering temperature from 900 °C to 1200 °C, where it peaks at 97.50% theoretical density. Further increase in the sintering temperature to 1300 °C leads to a fall in sintered density, when the decomposition of HA occurs, as has been confirmed using XRD for phase analysis [18,19]. Figure 9 illustrates the dependence of Vickers hardness on sintering temperature for the activation-derived hydroxyapatite. The steady increase in hardness is apparently due to the increase in sintered density up to 1200 °C.

Beyond 1200 °C, other calcium phosphate phases are formed, such as TCP, and therefore a lower hardness results [20].

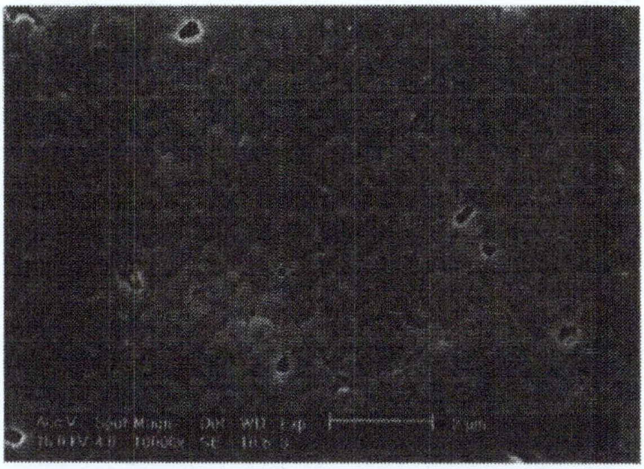

Fig. 7(a): SEM micrograph of polished natural surface of pellet derived from powders mechanically activated for 30 hours, ball-milled for 24 hours, isostatically pressed at 345 MPa and sintered at 1200 °C.

Fig. 7(b): SEM micrograph of fracture surface of pellet derived from powders mechanically activated for 30 hours, ball-milled for 24 hours, isostatically pressed at 345 MPa and sintered at 1200 °C.

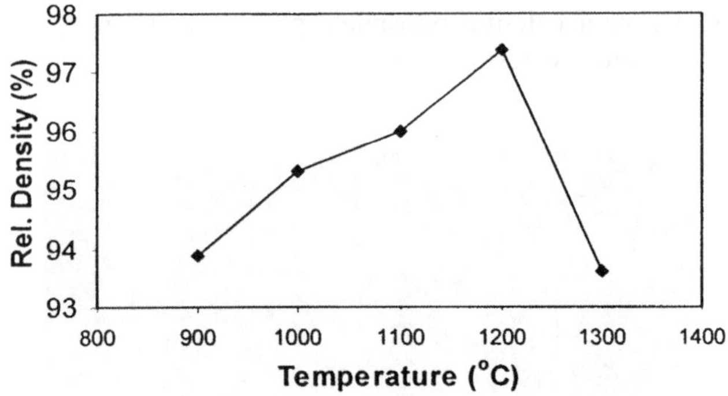

Fig. 8: Relative densities of HA derived from powders subjected to further ball-milling as a function of sintering temperature in the range of 900 °C to 1300 °C.

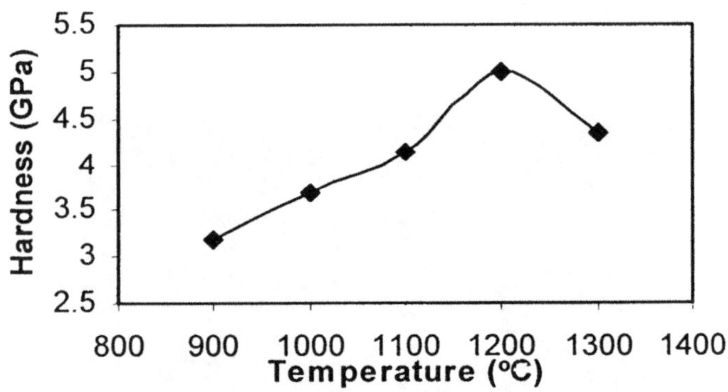

Fig. 9: Vickers Hardness as a function of sintering temperature for hydroxyapatite pellets isostatically pressed at 345 MPa.

CONCLUSIONS

Using calcium oxide (CaO) and brushite ($CaHPO_4.2H_2O$) as the starting powders, an ultrafine hydroxyapatite powder has been synthesized via a high-energy mechanical activation route. The formation of nanocrystalline hydroxyapatite was triggered in the powder mixture at 30 hours of mechanical activation. Calcination of the powder synthesized by 30 hours of mechanical activation at 800 °C lead to the formation of highly crystalline hydroxyapatite. This temperature is lower than what has been reported before for the starting powders used and is attributed to the completion of the reactions between the starting powders during mechanical activation. A maximum sintered density of 97.50% theoretical was observed at a sintering temperature of 1200 °C.

ACKNOWLEDGEMENTS

The authors are grateful to P.L. Chong of the School of Biological Science, for his help in taking the transmission electron micrographs. We would also like to thank Dr. J.M. Xue, G.K. Lim, and D.M. Wan for their help and discussions throughout the course of this project.

REFERENCES

1. A.S. Posner, in "*Phosphorous and Its Compounds, Vol. II*", edited by J.R. van Wazer Interscience, New York, (**1961**) 1429-1459
2. P. Ducheyne, L. Hench, A. Kagan, M.Martens, A. Burssens, J. Mulier, *J. Biomed. Mater. Res.* 14(**1980**) 225
3. A. Ravaglioli, A. Krajewski, "*Bioceramics: Materials, Properties, Applications*", Chapman & Hall, London (**1992**) 173-193 & 310-313
4. H. Aoki, "*Medical Applications of Hydroxyapatite*", Ishiyaku Euro-America, Tokyo (**1994**) 90-173
5. A. Deptula, W. Iada, T. Okak, *J. Non-Cryst. Sol.* 147/148 (**1992**) 537
6. Y. Fang, D.K. Agrawal, D.M. Roy, R. Roy, *Materials Letters* 23(**1995**) 147-151
7. C.H. Lin, C.W. Huang, S.C. Chang, *Mat. Res. Soc. Symp. Proc. Vol.* 346(**1994**) 237-241
8. M. Yoshimura, H. Suda, K. Okamoto, K. Ioku, *J. Mater. Sci.*, 29(**1994**) 3399-3402
9. J. Li, L. Hermansson, *Interceram.* 39(**1990**)
10. G.K. Lim, J. Wang, S.C. Ng, L.M. Gan, *Materials Letters* 28(**1996**) 431-436
11. M. Toriyama, S. Kawamura, *J. Ceram. Soc., Jpn. Int. Ed.* , 95(**1987**) 698-702

12. M. Toriyama, A. Ravaglioli, A. Krajewski, G. Celloti, A. Piancastelli, *J. Euro. Ceram. Soc.* 16(**1996**) 429-436.
13. H.P. Klug, L.E. Alexander, "*X-Ray Diffraction Procedures for Polycrystalline and Amorphous Materials*", Willey, New York (**1954**) 491-538
14. X. Yang, Z. Wang, *J. Mater. Chem.* 8(10) (**1998**) 2233-2237
15. M. Toriyama, S. Kawamura, Y. Ito, H. Nagae, *J. Ceram. Jpn. Int. Ed.* 97(5) (**1989**) 554-558
16. L. Lü, M. O. Lai, "*Mechanical Alloying*", Kluwer Academic Publisher, London (**1998**) 26-42
17. T. Kanazawa, "*Materials Science Monographs, 52: Inorganic Phosphate Materials*", Kodansha Elsevier, Tokyo (**1989**) 17
18. J. Zhou, X. Zhang, J. Chen, S. Zeng, K. De Groot, *J. Mater. Sci. Mater. Med.* 4(**1993**) 83
19. A. Tampieri, G. Celotti, F. Szontagh, E. Landi, *J. Mater. Sci. Mater. Med.* 8(**1997**) 29-37
20. M. Jarcho, C. H. Bolen, M. Thomas, J. Bobick, J. Kay, R. Doremus, *J. Mater. Sci.* **11**(1976) 2027

PREPARATION OF BIOMIMETIC HA PRECURSORS AT 37°C IN UREA- AND ENZYME UREASE-CONTAINING SYNTHETIC BODY FLUIDS

Defne Bayraktar and A. Cüneyt Taş *

Department of Metallurgical and Materials Engineering, Middle East Technical University, Ankara 06531, Turkey.

ABSTRACT

An important inorganic phase of synthetic bone applications, calcium hydroxyapatite (HA, $Ca_{10}(PO_4)_6(OH)_2$), was prepared as a single-phase and sub-micron bioceramic precursor powder. Carbonated HA precursors were synthesized from calcium nitrate tetrahydrate and di-ammonium hydrogen phosphate salts dissolved in "synthetic body fluid" (SBF) solutions, containing urea (H_2NCONH_2) and enzyme urease, under the biomimetic conditions of 37°C and pH 7.4, by using a novel chemical precipitation technique. These powders were also found to contain trace amounts of Na and Mg ions in them, intentionally incorporated by using SBF solutions, instead of pure water, during their synthesis. The characterization and chemical analysis of the synthesized biomimetic HA precursors were performed by scanning electron microscopy (SEM), powder X-ray diffraction (XRD), Fourier-transformed infra-red spectroscopy (FT-IR), and inductively-coupled plasma atomic emission spectroscopy (ICP-AES).

INTRODUCTION

Calcium hydroxyapatite (HA: $Ca_{10}(PO_4)_6(OH)_2$), the main inorganic component of the hard tissues in bones, is a member of "apatite" family of compounds. Biological apatites, which comprise the mineral phases of calcified tissues (enamel, dentin, and bone), slightly differ from pure HA in stoichiometry, composition and crystallinity, and in other physical and mechanical properties. They were usually observed [1] to be carbonate-substituted and calcium-deficient.

Synthetic body fluids (SBF) prepared in accord with the chemical analysis of human body fluid, with ion concentrations nearly equal to those of the inorganic constituents of human blood plasma, were first used by Kokubo, *et al.* [2], to prove the similarity between in vitro and in vivo behavior of certain glass-ceramic compositions. In these studies, the glass-ceramic samples were soaked in SBF solutions, and their surfaces were observed to be coated with a poorly crystallized calcium deficient and carbonate containing apatite, which was similar to bone apatite [3].

HA powders for bioceramic applications have generally been synthesized by using aqueous solutions. It is known [4] that calcium hydroxyapatite is the least soluble and the most stable compound of calcium phosphate phases in aqueous solutions at pH values

* *Present address: Max-Planck-Institut, Heisenbergstraße 5, D-70569, Stuttgart, Germany*

higher than 4.2. However, HA powders synthesized in highly alkaline media [5-10] were recognized by their relatively high thermal stability and phase purity even after high temperature (1100°-1300°C) sintering. Chemical synthesis of HA powders in neutral and/or slightly acidic aqueous media is known to be a more complicated and difficult task [7, 11]. This study [12] will focus on the determination of the experimental parameters of HA synthesis at the physiological pH (7.4) and temperature (37°C), in SBF solutions rich in urea and enzyme urease.

K. de Groot, *et al.* [8] studied the high-temperature characteristics of synthetic HA and reported that the synthetic HA with a Ca/P ratio near to 1.67 was only stable below 1200°C, when sintered in a dry or wet air atmosphere. It was claimed that beyond 1200°C, HA loses its OH^- groups gradually and transforms into oxyapatite ($Ca_{10}(PO_4)_6O$). When heated to 1450°C, oxyapatite was found [8] to dissociate into β-TCP, $Ca_2P_2O_7$ and $Ca_4P_2O_9$. On the other hand, Tas, *et. al.* [10] recently reported that pure HA powders prepared in distilled water may withstand, without decomposition, temperatures as high as 1300°C when heated for 6 h in a stagnant air atmosphere.

The surface properties and synthesis conditions of calcium hydroxyapatite, prepared by using pure water in highly alkaline medium, has previously been examined in different buffers [4, 6, 13] including the SBF; however, there is no published work, to our knowledge, on the "precipitation and formation" of calcium hydroxyapatite precursors in SBF solutions, containing urea and/or enzyme urease, at 37°C and pH of 7.4. The study presented here thus becomes the first systematic step taken in this specific field of "biomimetic" HA powder synthesis technology.

EXPERIMENTAL PROCEDURE

(1) Preparation of Synthetic Body Fluid (SBF)

SBF is known to be a metastable [3] buffer solution, and even a small, undesired variance in both of the preparation steps and the storage temperatures may drastically affect the phase purity and high-temperature stability of the produced HA powders, as well as the kinetics of the precipitation processes.

Merck (Darmstadt, Germany)-grade NaCl (99.5 %), $NaHCO_3$ (99.5 %), KCl (99.0 %), $Na_2HPO_4.2H_2O$ (99.5 %), $MgCl_2.6H_2O$ (98.0 %), Na_2SO_4, $(CH_2OH)_3CNH_2$ (99.2 %), $CaCl_2.2H_2O$ (99.0 %) and HCl (37 vol%, Carlo-Erba, Italy) were used in the preparation of the synthetic body fluids. SBF solutions were prepared [12] by dissolving appropriate quantities of the above chemicals in de-ionized water. Reagents were added, one by one after each was completely dissolved in 700 mL of water, in the order given in Table I.

A total of 40 mL of 1M HCl solution was consumed for pH adjustments during the preparation of SBF solutions. The 15 mL aliquot of this amount was added just before the addition of the 6th reagent, i.e., $CaCl_2.2H_2O$. The second portion of the HCl solution was used in the remainder of the titration process. Following the addition of the 8th

Table I. Chemical composition of SBF solutions *

Order	Reagent	Amount (gpl)
1	$NaCl$	6.547
2	$NaHCO_3$	2.268
3	KCl	0.373
4	$Na_2HPO_4.\ 2H_2O$	0.178
5	$MgCl_2.\ 6H_2O$	0.305
6	$CaCl_2.2H_2O$	0.368
7	Na_2SO_4	0.071
8	$(CH_2OH)_3CNH_2$	6.057

* _Patent Pending_, Turkish Patent Institute, Turkey, Appl. No: 99/00037, January 11, 1999.

reagent (tris(hydroxymethyl)-aminomethane), solution temperature was raised from the ambient to 37°C. This solution was then appropriately titrated with 1M HCl to the pH value of 7.4. During the titration process, the solution was also continuously diluted with consecutive additions of de-ionized water to make the final volume equal to 1 L.

The nominal, starting ion concentrations of the SBF solutions used in this study were matched more closely with those of "human plasma" than the ones given by Kokubo and his co-workers [2, 3]. The most significant differences of this study, as compared to the previous workers, in terms of "SBF ion concentrations" can be stated as follows: *(a)* the nominal, initial HCO_3^- ion concentration of SBF was increased from 4.2 mM to 27.0 mM which, thus, acquired exactly the same value with that of human plasma, *(b)* Cl^- ion concentration was decreased from 147.8 mM to 125.0 mM in the preparation recipe, whereas the Cl^- ion concentration of human plasma is 103.0 mM. This has solely been achieved by changing the 4th reagent of SBF preparation recipe from K-phosphate [2, 3] to Na-phosphate. The differences between the ion concentrations of our SBF solutions and those of human plasma are compared in Table II.

Table II. Ion concentrations of SBF solutions and human plasma

Ion	Kokubo, *et al.*[2,3](mM)	Present work (mM)	Human plasma(mM)
Na^+	142.0	142.0	142.0
Cl^-	147.8	125.0	103.0
HCO_3^-	4.2	27.0	27.0
K^+	5.0	5.0	5.0
Mg^{2+}	1.5	1.5	1.5
Ca^{2+}	2.5	2.5	2.5
HPO_4^{2-}	1.0	1.0	1.0
SO_4^{2-}	0.5	0.5	0.5

(2) Synthesis of HA Precursors in SBF Solutions

0.4 M $Ca(NO_3)_2.4H_2O$ (Riedel de-Haen, 99%, Germany) and 0.16 M $(NH_4)_2HPO_4$ (Merck, 99%, Germany) stock solutions were used in the precipitation experiments as the calcium and phosphate ion sources. 8 to 9.5 M urea solutions were prepared (by dissolving the urea powder in SBF) and then aged at 85°C overnight in a sealed glass jar, to ensure the decomposition of urea. The pH values of 9.5 M, "aged urea" solutions were measured as 9.3 at 37°C, prior to their use in powder synthesis. The enzyme urease (Merck, Lot No: 108489, 5 units/mg, Germany) was added, within the concentration range of 2.5 to 10 units/mL, into the precipitation solutions to establish [14] and accelerate the complete decompositon of urea at 37°C.

The precipitation scheme developed during the HA precursor synthesis experiments was given in the flowchart of Figure 1. For a total volume of 205 mL of SBF, according to Fig. 1, 0.4 mL of 1 gpl methyl cellulose stock solution was used as a dispersant. 410 mg of enzyme urease was dissolved in the above urea-containing SBF solutions to keep its initial concentration at the level of 10 units/mL. The pH values of the solutions were maintained [12] at the physiological level of 7.4 during the entire chemical precipitation experiments. The synthesized powders were then calcined in air over the temperature range of 300°-1600°C for 6 to 17 hours, following their drying at 80°C.

(3) Powder Characterization

The phase purity and the levels of crystallinity of the calcined HA powders were studied by powder X-ray diffraction (Model: D-Max/B, Rigaku Co., Tokyo, Japan) at the typical step size of 0.05° 2 θ and a count time of 1 s. A monochromated Cu-K_α tube operated at 40 kV and 20 mA was used for the generation of X-rays. All of the collected X-ray spectra were corrected for the shifts in the d-spacings by using pure silicon (Starck Inc., Germany) as an external standard. A least-squares unit cell refinement program [15] was used for the precise determination of crystallographic parameters of the synthesized powders. The further details of XRD analysis were described elsewhere [16].

Fourier-transformed infra-red spectroscopy (FT-IR) (Model: DX-510, Nicolet Co., WI, USA) was used in the wave number range of 4000-400 cm^{-1}. Experimental spectra of solid samples were obtained by preparing KBr pellets with a 3:97 (wt%) sample-to-KBr proportions.

(4) Chemical Analysis

Inductively-coupled plasma atomic emission spectroscopy (ICP-AES) (Model Plasma-1000, Perkin Elmer Co., London, UK) was used for the accurate chemical analysis of Na and Mg ions in the SBF-synthesized HA precursors (after being dissolved in acid solutions) which were believed to originate from the use of synthetic body fluids during the synthesis experiments.

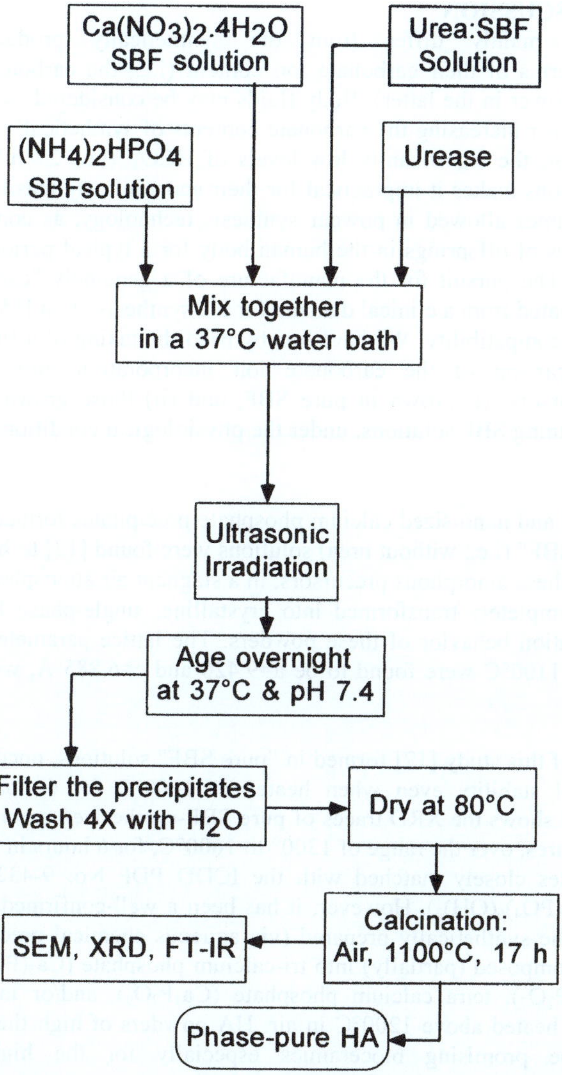

Fig. 1 **Process flowchart of precipitation route used in biomimetic HA synthesis**

RESULTS AND DISCUSSION

Biological apatites mainly differ from the synthetically produced calcium hydroxyapatites in terms of their carbonate ion content (i.e., the carbonate ion levels being incomparably lower in the latter). Body fluids may be considered as a biomimetic and plausible source for increasing the carbonate contents of synthetically prepared HA bioceramics. However, the significantly low levels of HCO_3^- (i.e., 27 mM) in human plasma or SBF solutions makes it impractical for their economically feasible use within the shorter "aging" times allowed in powder synthesis technology, as compared to the aging of natural bones of offsprings in the human body for a typical period of about "9 months + 10 days." The pursuit for the manufacture of a genuinely "carbonated" HA powder mainly originated from a clinical demand for the synthesis of an HA powder with improved in vivo biocompatibility. We have hereby tried the taking of a first systematic step into the comparison of the carbonate ion incorporation into the resultant hydroxyapatite precursors; (i) grown in pure SBF, and (ii) those grown in urea- and enzyme urease-containing SBF solutions, under the physiological conditions of 37°C and pH of 7.4.

The as-filtered, dried and nano-sized calcium phosphate precipitates formed at 37°C and pH of 7.4 via "pure SBF" (i.e., without urea) solutions were found [17] to be amorphous. Upon calcination of these amorphous precursors, in a stagnant air atmosphere, at 1100°C for 6 hours, they completely transformed into crystalline, single-phase HA. Figure 2 shows the crystallization behavior of these powders. The lattice parameters of the HA powders calcined at 1100°C were found to be a=9.420 and c=6.885 Å, with a unit cell volume of 529.04 $Å^3$.

The HA precursors of this study [17] formed in "pure SBF" solutions, uncommonly, had an excellent thermal stability even when heated at 1600°C for 6 hours in an air atmosphere. Figure 3 shows the XRD traces of pure SBF-synthesized precipitates heated at different temperatures, over the range of 1300° to 1600°C, for 6 hours in air. The XRD spectra of all samples closely matched with the ICDD PDF No: 9-432 for calcium hydroxyapatite ($Ca_{10}(PO_4)_6(OH)_2$). However, it has been a well-confirmed experimental fact [6, 8, 10] that the synthetically prepared (via aqueous chemical precipitation) HA powders usually decomposed (partially) into tri-calcium phosphate ($Ca_3(PO_4)_2$), calcium pyrophosphate ($Ca_2P_2O_7$), tetra calcium phosphate ($Ca_4P_2O_9$), and/or into oxyapatite ($Ca_{10}(PO_4)_6O$) when heated above 1200°C in air. HA powders of high thermal stability are expected to be promising bioceramics especially for the high-temperature applications, such as plasma-spraying.

Biomimetic HA powders of the present study also contained trace amounts of other inorganic ions, provided by SBF. ICP-AES analysis performed on representative 1200°C-calcined samples indicated that these HA powders had 1500 ppm Mg and 160 ppm Na. Na^+ and Mg^{2+} ions, originated from the use of SBF solutions during precipitation, were believed to incorporate themselves in the crystal structure of calcium hydroxyapatite. The CO_3^{2-} ions are known [1] to substitute, in part, the OH^- sites, and again, in part the PO_4^{3-} groups of the HA structure. On the other hand, Mg^{2+} ions were claimed [1] to replace the Ca^{2+} sites of the HA structure. We also believe that the Na^+ ions might have

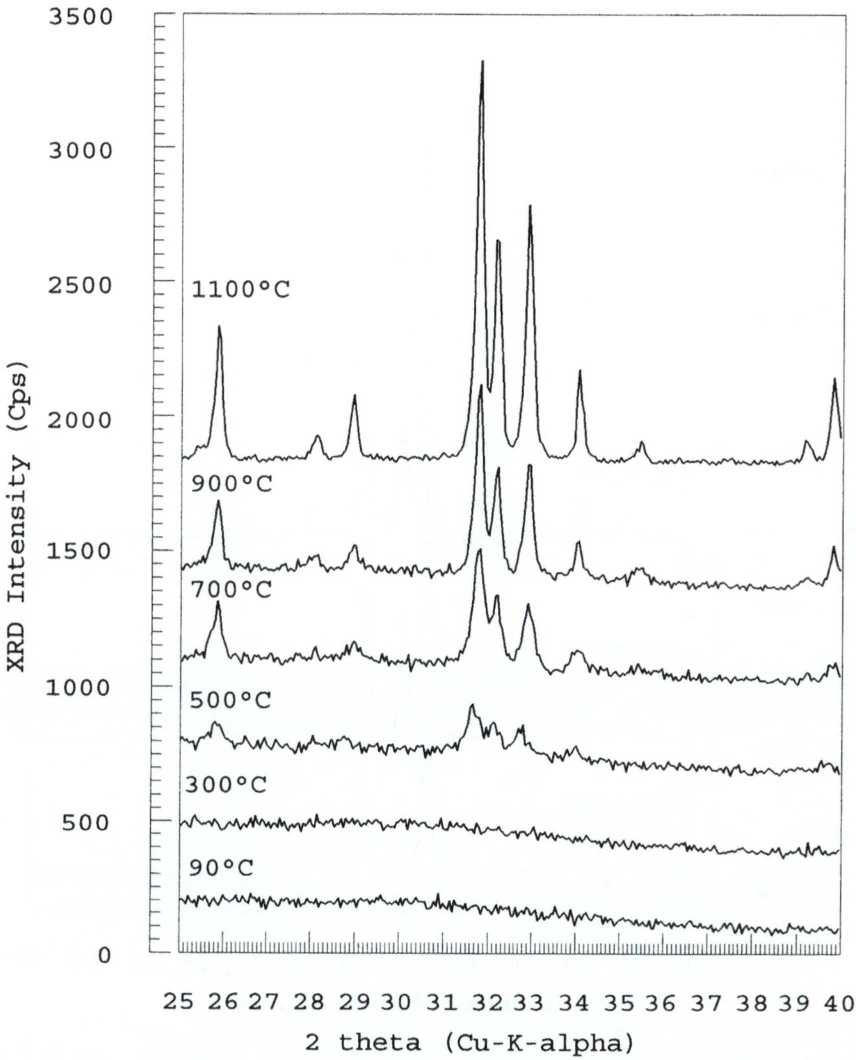

Fig. 2 Crystallization behavior of SBF-synthesized amorphous HA precursors

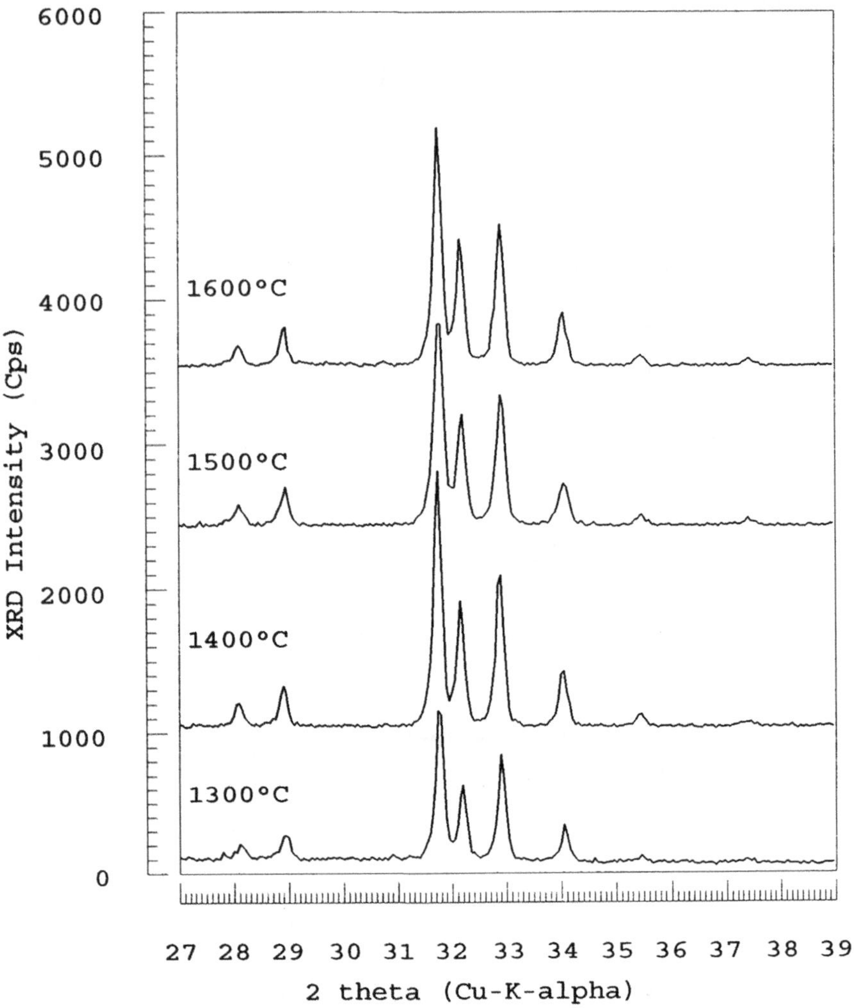

Fig. 3 XRD spectra of SBF-synthesized HA precursors after heating at different temperatures (1300°-1600°C, 6 h, air)

placed themselves nearby the OH^- sites (close to the P-bonded oxygens), and hence, caused a reduction in the extent of de-hydroxylation at the significantly high calcination temperatures of this study.

The FT-IR spectra of SBF-synthesized HA precursors were given in Figure 4. The top spectrum of this figure belonged to pure SBF-grown (i.e., SBF solutions without urea/urease) HA precipitates, after 6 hours of calcination at 700°C in air. The CO_3^{2-} ion peaks, at 2368-2361 (combination of $\nu_2 + \nu_3$), 1467-1412 and 878 cm^{-1}, were clearly visible. As the calcination temperature increased, the FT-IR peaks of the CO_3^{2-} totally disappeared. The OH^- stretching vibration was observed at 3571 cm^{-1} and the OH^- bending vibration was recorded at 635 cm^{-1}. The PO_4 bands [18] were detected at 470 (ν_2), 570 and 603 (ν_4), 962 (ν_1), 1045 and 1096 (ν_3) cm^{-1}. The bottom FT-IR spectrum of Figure 4 was obtained from the powder synthesis experiments which used the urea- and enzyme urease-containing SBF solutions. The significant qualitative presence of carbonate ions in HA structure was again clearly apparent.

The morphology of these biomimetic HA precursors were observed by the SEM micrographs given in Figure 5. The micrograph given in Figure 5(a) showed the sub-micron (with an average value of 0.25 μm) particles of as-filtered biomimetic powders after drying at 90°C. The particles shown were first ultrasonically dispersed in isopropyl alcohol (5 mg powder in 10 mL alcohol) and then a drop of the formed dispersion was evaporated on a clean glass substrate, prior to SEM study. The micrograph given in Figure 5(b), on the other hand, showed the morphology of the same powders after being heated at 1150°C for 12 hours, in the form of a loose powder compact in an alumina crucible. The investigation of the sintering behavior of such powders would be important for the production of densified bioceramic prostheses and parts. A further set of decisive carbon analysis would, however, be required for a quantitative determination of the amounts of CO_3^{2-} ions present in such samples.

The use of SBF solutions and the addition of enzyme urease to the SBF solutions containing urea were both attempted for the first time, in the present study, for the synthesis of biomimetic, carbonated HA precursors. In the HA synthesis practices which used the starting chemicals of $Ca(NO_3)_2.4H_2O$ and $(NH_4)_2HPO_4$, it was known that the if the synthesis medium was pure water, then the solution pH values must be in the alkaline region [6-11]. On the other hand, in the case of using SBF, the pH value needed for HA synthesis decreases [12, 17, 19] considerably. In combination with the initial presence of spontaneously formed seed crystals [12, 17, 19] in precipitation solutions, the high ionic strength of the precipitation medium (provided by SBF) played an important role in inducing the formation of pure calcium hydroxyapatite precursor phase that would otherwise, normally, not nucleate at such a low pH value of 7.4. Following the addition of the enzyme urease into the precipitation solutions, the pH values have changed as shown in Figure 6. (Without the addition of enzyme urease into the same solutions, the plots would look like horizontal, straight lines.) When the enzyme concentration was kept at the initial, nominal level of 2.5 units/mL, the synthesized powders were consisted of two phases, i.e., a mixture of HA (20%) and $Ca_3(PO_4)_2$ (20%). However, when the enzyme concentration was increased to 10 units/mL, the solution pH value was observed

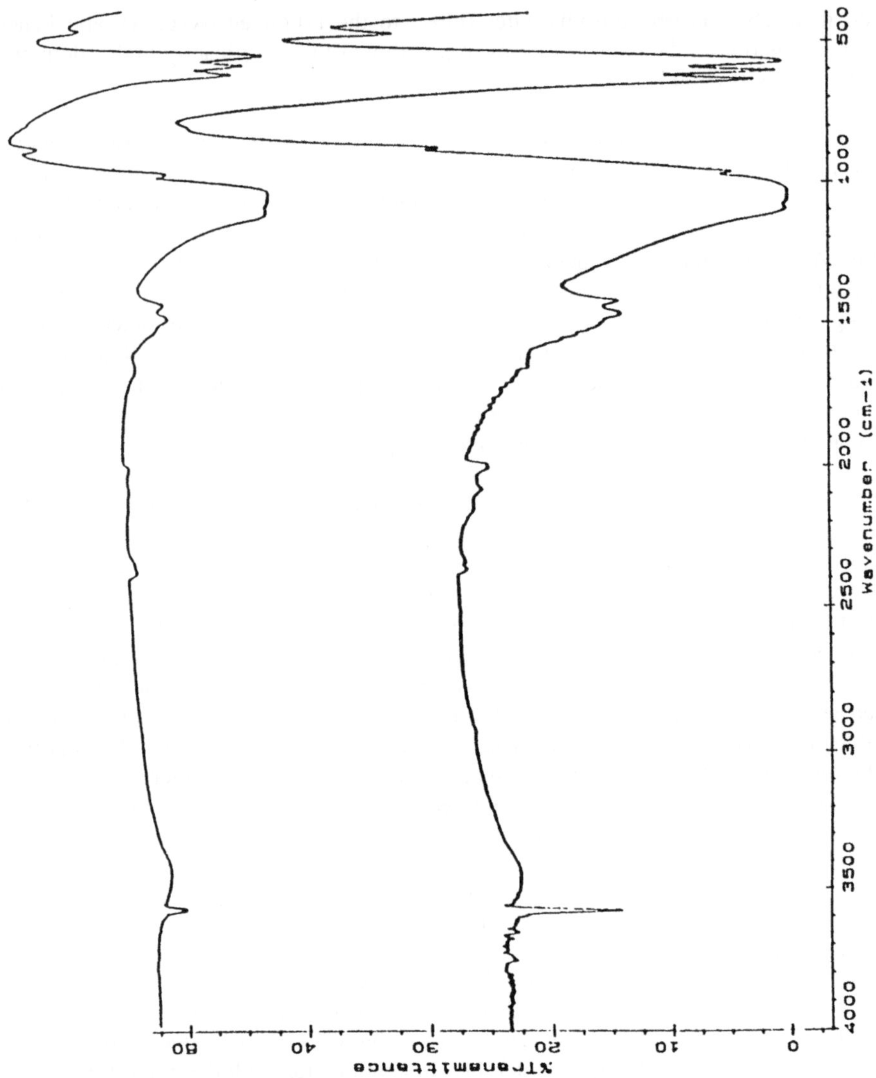

Fig. 4 FT-IR spectra of SBF-synthesized HA precursors (*Top*: in pure SBF, *Bottom*: in urea- and enzyme urease-containing SBF, samples heated at 700°C in air for 6 h)

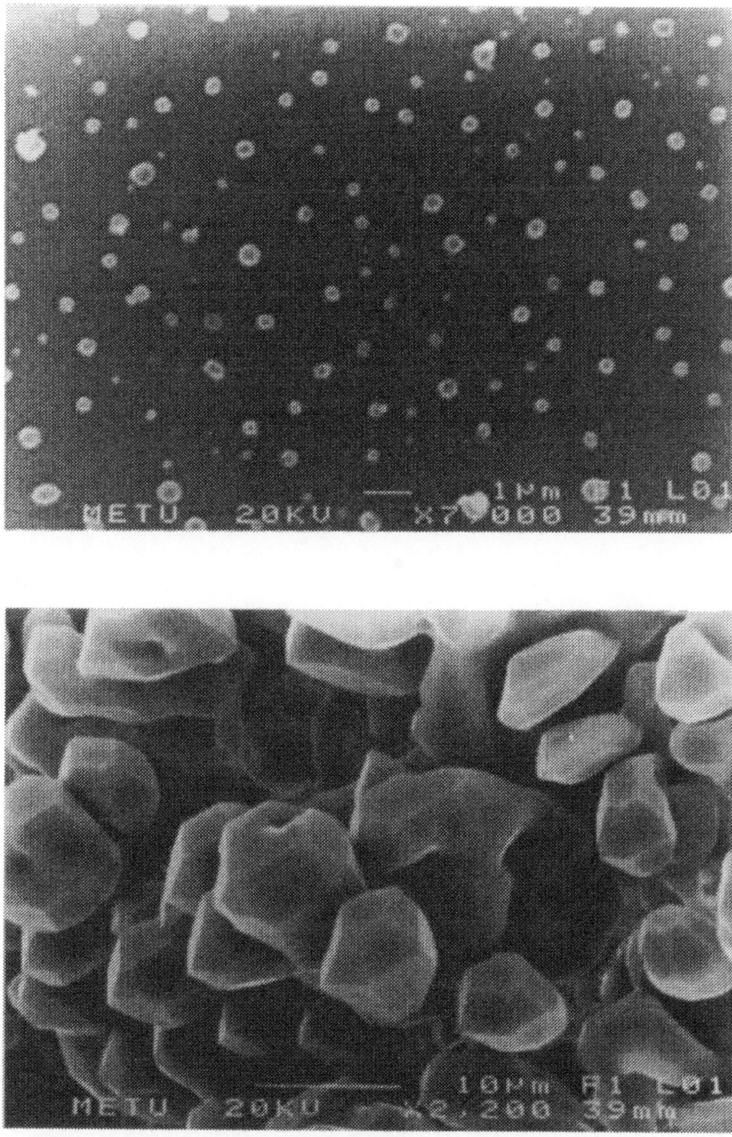

Fig. 5 SEM micrographs of SBF-synthesized (urea/urease) HA precursors, (*Top*: 90°C, *Bottom*: 1150°C)

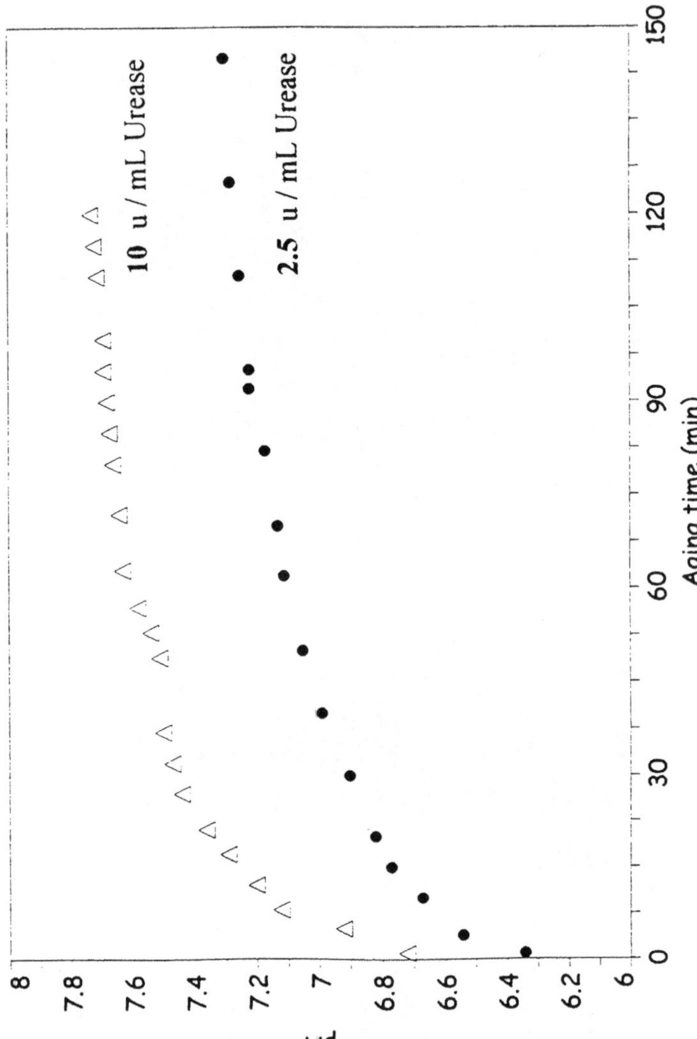

Fig. 6 pH control provided by the enzyme urease (at two different concentrations) in urea-ctg. SBF solutions during Ca-phosphate powder precipitation at 37°C

to rise to the vicinity of 7.4, in about the first half hour of aging at 37°C. The powders obtained at this concentration of urease were found to be single phase HA after calcination at 1100°C. The biomimetic pH control (around the neighborhood of pH 7.4) in urea-containing synthetic body fluids have thus been shown to be achievable, at 37°C, by the addition of the enzyme urease in appropriate amounts (8-10 units/mL).

CONCLUSIONS

Chemically homogeneous, single-phase calcium hydroxyapatite (HA) precursors have been synthesized by a novel chemical precipitation technique via synthetic body fluid solutions (either pure or urea/enzyme urease-containing), at the physiological conditions of pH 7.4 and 37°C, with dissolved calcium nitrate tetrahydrate and di-ammonium hydrogen phosphate salts in appropriate amounts. The produced powders were shown to be carbonated and to have unprecedented phase stability even when heated at 1600°C, for 6 hours, in a stagnant air atmosphere. Biomimetic HA powders were also shown to have small amounts of other inorganic ions, provided and incorporated into the HA structure by the SBF solutions used during synthesis. ICP analysis performed on calcined powders indicated that the HA powders of this study had 1500 ppm Mg and 160 ppm Na. Enzyme urease when added in proper amounts into the urea-containing synthetic body fluids used for HA precursor synthesis was shown to supply a plausible pH control required for the achievement of biomimetic conditions.

REFERENCES

1. L. L. Hench and J. Wilson, "An Introduction to Bioceramics," World Scientific, London, 1993, pp. 8, 146, 331, 335.

2. T. Kokubo, "Surface Chemistry of Bioactive Glass Ceramics," *J. Non-Crystal. Sol.*, **120**, 138-51 (1990).

3. C. Ohtsuki, T. Kokubo, and T. Yamamuro, "Mechanism of HA Formation on CaO-SiO_2-P_2O_5 Glasses in Simulated Body Fluid," *J. Non-Crystal. Sol.*, **143**, 84-92 (1992).

4. C. P. A. T. Klein, J. M. A. De Blieck-Hogerworst, J. G. C. Wolke, K. De Groot, "Studies of Solubility of Different Calcium Phosphate Ceramic Particles In Vitro," *Biomaterials*, **11**, 509-12 (1990).

5. M. Jarcho, C. H. Bolen, M. B. Thomas, J. Babock, J. F. Kay, and R. H. Doremus, "Hydroxyapatite Synthesis and Characterization in Dense Polycrystalline Form," *J. Mat. Sci.*, **11**, 2027-35 (1976).

6. M. Asada, Y. Miura, A. Osaka, K. Oukami, and S. Nakamura, "Hydroxyapatite Crystal Growth on Calcium Hydroxyapatite Ceramics," *J. Mat. Sci.*, **23**, 3202-5 (1988).

7. E. Ebrahimpour, M. Johnson, C. F. Richardson, and G. H. Nancollas, "The Characterization of HA Precipitation," *J. Coll. Int. Sci.*, **159**, 158-63 (1993).

8. J. Zhou, X. Zhang, J. Chen, S. Zeng, and K. De Groot, "High Temperature Characteristics of Synthetic Hydroxyapatite," *J. Mat. Sci.: Mat. in Med.*, **4**, 83-5 (1993).

9. S. Lazic, "Microcrystalline Hydroxyapatite Formation from Alkaline Solutions," *J. Cryst. Growth*, **147**, 147-54 (1995).

10. A. C. Tas, F. Korkusuz, M. Timucin, and N. Akkas, "An Investigation of the Chemical Synthesis and High-Temperature Sintering Behaviour of Calcium Hydroxyapatite (HA) and Tricalcium Phosphate (TCP) Bioceramics," *J. Mat. Sci.: Mat. in Med.*, **8**, 91-6 (1997).
11. H. E. L. Madsen and G. Thodvadarson, "Precipitation of Calcium Phosphate from Moderately Acid Solutions," *J. Cryst. Growth*, **66**, 369-76 (1984).
12. A. C. Tas, "Biomimetic Synthesis of Carbonated Calcium Hydroxyapatite Powders at 37°C with Urea- or Enzyme Urease-containing Synthetic Body Fluids," Patent Pending, No: 99/00037, Turkish Patent Institute, Ankara, Turkey, January 11, 1999.
13. L. Yubao, C. P. A. T. Klein, Z. Xingdong, K. De Groot, "Formation of a Bone Apatite-Like Layer on the Surface of Porous HA Ceramics," *Biomaterials*, **15**, 835-40 (1994).
14. R. E. Simpson, C. Habeger, A. Rabinovich and J. H. Adair, "Enzyme-Catalyzed Inorganic Precipitation of Aluminum Basic Sulfate," *J. Am. Ceram. Soc.*, **81**, 1377-79 (1998).
15. D. E. Appleman and H. T. Evans, "Least-Squares and Indexing Software for XRD Data," U.S. Geological Survey, Computer Contribution No.20, U.S. National Technical Information Service, Document PB-216188 (1973).
16. N. Kivrak and A. C. Tas, "Synthesis of Calcium Hydroxyapatite-Tricalcium Phosphate (HA-TCP) Composite Bioceramic Powders and Their Sintering Behavior," *J. Am. Ceram. Soc.*, **81**, 2245-52 (1998).
17. F. A. Simsek, "Chemical Preparation of Calcium Hydroxyapatite (HA) in Synthetic Body Fluids at 37°C and Its Use in Chemical Coating of Titanium and Stainless Steel Strips," M.Sc. Thesis, (Thesis Supervisors: A. C. Tas and H. O. Pamuk), Middle East Technical University, July 1997.
18. N. Pleshka, A. Boskey, and R. Mendelsohn, "Novel Infrared Spectroscopic Method on the Determination of Crystallinity of Hydroxyapatite Minerals," *Biophys. J.*, **60**, 786-93 (1991).
19. F. A. Simsek, H. O. Pamuk, and A. C. Tas, "Synthesis of HA Bioceramic Powders at 37°C by using Synthetic Body Fluids," 99th Annual Meeting of The American Ceramic Society, Bioceramics Symposium, Cincinnati, Ohio, USA, May 1997.

PHYSICAL CHARACTERISTICS OF SINTERED HYDROXYAPATITE

T. P. Hoepfner and E. D. Case
Materials Science and Mechanics Department
Michigan State University
East Lansing, MI 48824

ABSTRACT

Hydroxyapatite is the principal inorganic component of bone, and is an implant material for skeletal reconstruction. Hydroxyapatite is a single phase ceramic with a reported large thermal expansion anisotropy. Large thermal expansion anisotropy is known to cause microcracking upon cooling in ceramics, and such microcracking is a strong function of the grain size. The discussion focuses on the relationship between microcracking in sintered hydroxyapatite and properties such as hardness and fracture toughness.

INTRODUCTION

Hydroxyapatite (HAP) is of considerable interest as a bio-implant material, either by itself or as part of a composite. However, for ceramics such as HAP, material properties, including the elastic modulus, thermal expansion, thermal conductivity, and thermal diffusivity are strongly affected by microcracking, and the values of these properties change significantly if microcracking exists [1]. In this context, microcracks are cracks with a very small aspect ratio (crack opening displacement/crack length).

Three mechanisms by which microcracks are induced in brittle materials are: (1) thermal expansion anisotropy or TEA, (2) thermal expansion mismatch between different crystallographic phases, and (3) rapid, displacive phase transitions [1]. TEA refers to the fact that for non-cubic crystalline lattices, the thermal expansion along different crystallographic axis differ from axis to axis. The thermal expansion anisotropy (TEA) causes the grains to shrink at different rates in different directions, for example, during cooling, and these differing rates of thermal contraction create stresses between adjacent grains. The greater the TEA, the greater the stress [1]. Stresses between adjacent grains arising from differing thermal expansion coefficients of differing phases and from a rapid phase transition also can induce microcracking. However, in this study x-ray diffraction measurements indicate a minimal second phase formation in the HAP, which indicates that among the microcracking mechanisms discussed above, TEA is the mechanism most likely to be operative.

In this study a commercially available hydroxyapatite powder has been sintered at temperatures between 1300°C and 1400°C (Table 1), resulting in a range of mean grain sizes between about 1.5 and 7 microns in the densified specimens (Table 2). The variation in the fracture toughness as a function of grain size may be indicative of microcracking in the HAP, but further studies are needed to clarify this point.

BACKGROUND

Hydroxyapatite is one member of the class of minerals known as apatites having the general chemical formula $Ca_5(PO_4)_3X$, where X denotes either $(OH)_2$, F_2, or Cl. Hydroxyapatite is generally found in a hexagonal crystal structure with the space group $P6_3/m$ [2]. Other researchers have observed the precipitation of hydroxyapatite into a monoclinic structure having space group $P2_1/b$, which in turn has phase change to the hexagonal structure at 211°C [3]. The room temperature hydroxyapatite lattice parameters are: a = 0.9421 nm, b = 2a, c = 0.98814 nm, and γ =120 ° [2].

The hexagonal symmetry of HAP leads to an anisotropy in the thermal expansion coefficient. However, differing values exist in the literature for the thermal expansion as a function of crystallographic direction. The reported thermal expansion coefficients along the crystallographic axes vary from α_a = 14.1 $x10^{-6}/^{o}C$ and α_c = 21.9$x10^{-6}/^{o}C$ [4] to α_a = 11.8 $x10^{-6}/^{o}C$ and α_c = 11.4$x10^{-6}/^{o}C$ [5]. Using these two papers [4, 5], the resulting differences in the thermal expansion coefficients, $\Delta\alpha$, along the crystallographic axis is then either 7.8 $x10^{-6}/^{o}C$ [4] or 0.4 $x10^{-6}/^{o}C$ [5]. Thus, unfortunately the literature is ambiguous in terms of the magnitude of the TEA, where a thermal expansion of 7.8 $x10^{-6}/^{o}C$ would correspond to a high value of TEA (indicating a relatively high tendency for microcracking), while a TEA of 0.4 $x10^{-6}/^{o}C$ is a low value of TEA (indicating a relatively low tendency for microcracking) [1].

Sintering hydroxyapatite (HAP) can lead to the partial thermal decomposition of HAP into tricalcium phosphate (TCP) and/or tetracalcium phosphate. The thermal decomposition is accomplished in two steps, (a) dehydroxylation and (b) decomposition [2, 6, 7, 8]. Dehydroxylation to oxyhydroxyapatite (OHA) proceeds by the fully reversible reaction [2,6]

$$Ca_{10}(PO_4)_6(OH)_2 \rightarrow Ca_{10}(PO_4)_6(OH)_{2-2x}O_x + xH_2O_{gas} \quad (1)$$

at temperatures from about 850^{0}C to 900^{0}C. The decomposition to TCP and tetracalcium phosphate occurs at temperatures greater than 900^{0}C by the reaction

$$Ca_{10}(PO_4)_6\,(OH)_2 \rightarrow 2Ca_3\,(PO_4)_2 + Ca_4P_2O_9 + H_2O_{gas} \qquad (2)$$

Since both the dehydroxylation and decomposition reactions include water vapor as a product, the rates for these reactions depend on the partial pressure of H_2O in the furnace atmosphere. The decomposition reactions (equations 1 and 2) allow one to control the secondary phase formation during sintering by controlling the sintering atmosphere. The literature [6, 9, 10] shows a great variation of secondary phase formation in HAP for similar sintering conditions. In this study, an x-ray diffraction study was included to determine the extent of second phase formation.

Thus, sintered HAP specimens are subject to microcracking due to both the inherent thermal expansion anisotropy (TEA) of the crystalline lattice and to differing crystallographic phases that can form during processing. Microcracking in turn can lead to changes in material properties such as thermal expansion [1], thermal diffusivity and thermal conductivity [1, 11]. Two studies in the literature [6, 12] indicate that HAP may in fact be subject to microcracking, but the data is not definitive in either study. Kijima and Tsutsumi [12] measured thermal diffusivity and thermal conductivity for the temperature interval from room temperature to 727 ^{0}C for sintered HAP specimens having a volume fraction porosity of 0.6 percent to 6.6 percent, with grain sizes ranging from 0.8 microns to 11.5 microns. The thermal conductivity and diffusivity increased as a function of grain size in the same way as would be expected from non-microcracked materials [12]. However, if all of the HAP specimens were microcracked and no diffusive crack healing occurred in the heating between room temperature and 727^{0}C, undetected microcrack population may have existed in the HAP specimens.

In another study of HAP, Royer et al. [6] observed a decline in the flexural strength HAP specimens as a function of increasing grain size for grain sizes greater than 0.9 microns. Royer et al. attributed the strength drop to the Petch-Hall relation for flexural strength, σ_f, versus grain size, g, namely that $\sigma_f = B(g)^{-1/2}$ where B is a constant. Royer's data is consistent both with Petch-Hall behavior [6] and with microcracking in the material [1], so Royer's results are not definitive with respect to microcracking in HAP. Halouani et al. [13] observed a drop in fracture strength and fracture toughness for hot-pressed HAP specimens having average grain sizes greater than 0.4 microns. Halouani et al. [13] attributed the decline in strength and toughness to microcracking due to TEA.

In order to interpret experimental measurements on materials whose properties may be affected by microcracking, as is the case for Kijima and Tsutsumi's study of thermal conductivity and thermal diffusivity [12] and Royer et al.'s study of strength and fracture toughness [6], it is helpful to have a theoretical framework that address the material properties that one would expect to govern the onset and severity of microcracking. For microcracking due to thermal expansion anisotropy, Cleveland and Bradt [14] give the following criterion for the critical grain size for microcracking, g_{cr}, where

$$g_{cr} = k\gamma_f / E(\Delta T \Delta\alpha)^2 \qquad (3)$$

and k is a constant based on the grain geometry, γ_f is the fracture surface energy, E is Young's modulus, $\Delta\alpha$ is the maximum difference in the thermal expansion coefficients along the crystallographic axes and ΔT is the difference between the sintering temperature and room temperature. For grains sizes above the critical grain size, microcracking occurs, while for grain sizes below the critical grain size, no microcracking occurs. As the grain size increases above g_{cr}, the severity of microcracking increases [1]. Thus, the question of the onset of microcracking is very much connected to the magnitude of $\Delta\alpha$, the difference in thermal expansion along the crystallographic axes. Since at least one study [4] reports a relatively high value of $\Delta\alpha$ ($7.8 \times 10^{-6}/^{o}C$) for HAP, it may be the case that HAP does microcrack, which could in term affect properties of interest for bio-implant materials, such as elastic modulus and strength.

EXPERIMENTAL PROCEDURE

The calcium hydoxapatite powder used in this study was specified by the vendor (Cerac Inc., Specialty Inorganics, Milwaukee, WI) as 99 percent pure. The powder, with no added binder, was pressed in a cylindrical hardened steel die at 6.54 MPa. Prior to pressing the specimens, the die was cleaned with acetone and no die lubricants were used. The as-pressed specimens were disks 5.095 cm in diameter and 3-4 cm thick depending on the mass of hydroxyapatite powder used (8 g, 10g, or 12 g).

In order to obtain sintered HAP having a range of grain sizes, the green specimens were fired in an electric tube furnace (Thermtec, Lenton Thermal Designs) at 1300° or 1400° C for 2-11 hours using a heating and cooling rate of 10°C/minute. After the specimens were sintered, density measurements were made using Archimedes method in distilled water. The average grain sizes of the sintered hydroxyapatite specimens were calculated using the linear intercept method on SEM micrographs of polished and etched specimen surfaces. More than 200 intercepts per micrograph were evaluated. A stereographic projection factor of 1.0 was used in the calculations.

Three different tests were performed on the sintered HAP specimens: (1) x-ray diffraction, in order to determine the phases present in the densified specimens, (2) Vickers indentation tests in order to obtain hardness and fracture toughness data, (3) thermal expansion, in order to determine whether the sintered HAP specimens exhibited differing thermal expansion behavior as a function of grain size that might be indicative of a microcracked material. For the x-ray analysis, specimens approximately 3 mm x 3 mm x 2 mm were cut from the sintered HAP disk-shaped specimens using a low speed diamond saw. Powdered HAP specimens for x-ray analysis were then prepared from the sintered HAP specimens by crushing and grinding the specimens in a porcelain crucible. The powder was then pressed into a deep-well x-ray mount fabricated from a glass microscope slide. Using a Scintag 2000 x-ray diffractometer and CuK_{α} radiation, diffraction angles between 25 and 36 degrees 2Θ were examined since this 2Θ range includes the most intense x-ray diffraction peaks from HAP and the HAP decomposition products, α and β (TCP) and tetracalcium phosphate [2].

Specimens approximately 5 mm x 5 mm x 2 mm were cut from the as-sintered HAP disks for the indentation study. From 7 to 10 Vickers indentation cracks were induced on the polished faces of the specimens using loads of 2.94 N, 4.9 N, and 9.8 N with a 10 second loading time and a 70 micron/second loading speed. Indentations that included visible spalling were not included in the data analysis.

For the thermal expansion measurements on HAP, bar-shaped specimens approximately 10 mm x 5 mm x 3 mm were cut from the disk specimens using a slow speed diamond saw. Opposing specimen faces were ground approximately parallel using 600 grit silicon carbide grit. The expansion data was collected using a thermomechanical analyzer (DuPont Instruments, Model 943), programmed to heat the specimen at 10°C/minute to 800°C and then hold at 800°C for 0, 10, 20, 30, or 60 minutes.

In order to determine the accuracy of the thermal expansion measurements, additional thermal expansion measurements were performed on a "standard" material, namely polycrystalline alumina specimens. The polycrystalline α-alumina specimens were obtained by sintering a high-purity alumina powder (AKP30, Sumitomo Corp.) for 1 hour at 1500°C yielding an average grain size of approximately 10 microns. Since α-alumina does not undergo stoichiometry or crystallographic changes upon heating in air, it is often used as a reference material in thermophysical measurements, such as in differential thermal analysis (DTA) procedures. From the sintered alumina billet, two specimens, one approximately 11 mm x 5 mm x 3 mm and the other about

13 mm x 5 mm x 3 mm was cut using a low speed diamond saw. The alumina specimens' thermal expansion was measured using the same thermomechanical analyzer (DuPont Instruments, Model 943) used for the thermal expansion measurements of the HAP specimens. The alumina was heated at a nominal rate of 10°C/minute to 800°C and with no hold time.

RESULTS AND DISCUSSION

For both the as-received HAP powder and for a representative sampling of the sintered hydroxyapatite specimens, all x-ray diffraction (XRD) peaks except one corresponded to the HAP phase (Figure 1). The one non-HAP peak corresponded to the most intense tetra-calcium phosphate peaks, which were found near a 2θ value of 29.5^{O} for specimens 8 and 12 (Tables 1 and 2). Thus, based on the XRD data, the tetra-calcium phosphate was the only second phase detectable by x-ray diffraction in the sintered HAP included in this study, and on the one occasion that tetra-calcium phosphate was detected, it was a minor phase. Thus if microcracking occurred in the HAP, thermal expansion anisotropy is a more likely mechanism than thermal expansion mismatch between differing phases.

Table 1 gives the processing parameters, density, and grain size for the HAP specimens sintered in this study. The average grain size increased from about 1.5 microns to 6.8 microns as the sintering time/temperature increased (Table 1). The hardness and toughness of the sintered HAP specimens were calculated from the Vickers indentation data using equations 4 and 5. The hardness, H, is related to the Vickers indentation diagonal length 2a by the relationship [15]

$$H = P / 2a^2 \tag{4}$$

where P is the applied Vickers indentation load. For Vickers indentation cracks in a brittle material, the mode I fracture toughness, K_{IC}, may be estimated by

$$K_{IC} = A\,(E/H)^{1/2} P c^{-3/2} \tag{5}$$

where the dimensionless calibration constant A equals 0.016 [15], E is the elastic modulus, H is the hardness calculated in equation 4, c is half the indentation crack length, and P is the applied indentation load. For the purpose of calculating K_{IC}, E was taken as 115 GPa [16].

The measured hardness of the sintered HAP specimens tended to increase as a function of grain size (Figure 2), and the toughness of the sintered specimens decreased as the grain size increased (Figure 3). The increasing hardness may be

Table I. Sintering data for hydroxyapatite specimens

Sample	Temp. ^{0}C	Time hours	Density g/cm^2	Grain Size x10^{-6} m
1	1300	1		
2	1300	1.25		1.51
3	1300	0.75		1.98
4	1300	1.5		2.07
5	1300	1.75	2.883	2.14
6	1300	4	2.920	2.32
7	1400	2	3.049	5.65
8	1400	4	3.060	7.44
9	1300	5	2.966	5.93
10	1300	7	2.953	5.93
11	1300	9	2.980	6.73
12	1300	11	2.974	6.80

Table II. Hardness and Toughness data of hydroxyapatite specimens

Sample	Density g/cm^2	Grain Size x10^{-6} m	Hardness GPa	Std dev. GPa	Toughness MPa m$^{1/2}$	Std dev. MPa m$^{1/2}$
1			3.543	0.274	1.125	0.266
2		1.51	3.333	0.248	1.233	0.238
3		1.98	2.792	0.234	1.466	0.231
4		2.07	3.758	0.432	1.017	0.294
5	2.883	2.14	3.774	0.515	1.006	0.187
6	2.920	2.32	3.326	0.281	1.209	0.204
7	3.049	5.65	4.816	0.551	0.794	0.259
8	3.060	7.44				
9	2.966	5.93				
10	2.953	5.93	3.671	0.150	0.833	0.354
11	2.980	6.73				
12	2.974	6.80	4.428	0.351	0.701	0.144

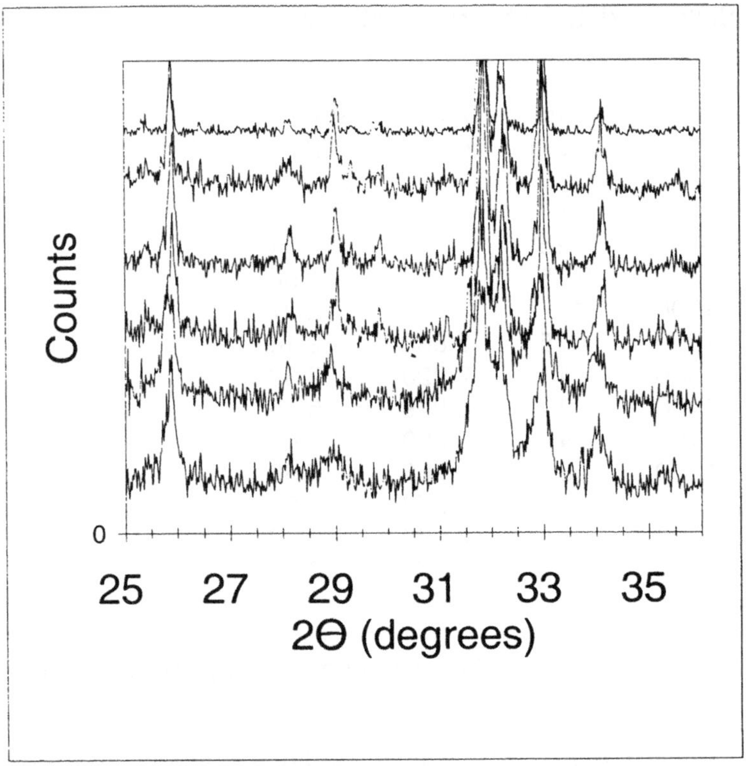

Figure 1 X-ray diffraction data for hydroxyapatite. Unsintered powder at bottom ascending to sintered specimens 6,7,8,10 and 12.

a grain size/mass density effect, rather than a microcracking effect. For example, the hardness of oxide and non-oxide ceramics tends to decrease as a porosity increases [17 - 19]. The trend of hardness as a function of grain size is less straightforward, as discussed in a review by Rice et al. [17], since the hardness tends to decrease with grain size for small grain sizes then go through a minimum at intermediate grain sizes, and increase for with increasing grain size for large grain sizes.

However, the observed fracture toughness (Figure 3) was somewhat lower than the values observed in the literature for small-grained HAP [6], which indicate that the decrease in fracture toughness with increasing grain size observed in this study may be a microcracking effect. No indication of a plateau in toughness values at small grain sizes was observed (Figure 3), which would be consistent with the condition that all specimens in this study had grain sizes larger than the critical grain size, g_{cr}, where an increasing grain size might lead to a monotonically decreasing fracture toughness. As reviewed by Rice [20], the fracture toughness values can go through a maximum as grain size increases, but this effect is often associated with microcracking, where a decreasing fracture toughness indicates that the grain size is larger than g_{cr}. Thus the observed decrease in fracture toughness with grain size (Figure 3) may indicate that for all of the specimens included in this study (Table 1), the grain size exceeds g_{cr}, but additional fracture toughness measurements are needed which include grain sizes smaller than g_{cr} for HAP.

During the thermal expansion measurements (Figures 4 and 5) the HAP specimens were heated to 800°C followed by soak times varying between zero and 60 minutes. The thermal expansion as a function of temperature was very similar for the entire range of grain sizes included in this experiment. The thermal expansion data for both the HAP (Figures 4 and 5) and alumina (Figure 6) were smoothed by moving average over 5 consecutive data points, that is, the thermal expansion α_i at temperature T_i was determined by the average $(\alpha_{i-2} + \alpha_{i-1} + \alpha_i + \alpha_{i+1} + \alpha_{i+2})/5$. Subsequently, the subscript "i" is incremented by one, and the "smoothed" value for the next thermal expansion point is again determined by averaging over 5 consecutive data points. Although the thermal expansion curves (Figures 4 and 5) do not show significant changes with grain size, the grain size range included in this study is relatively limited, in part do the phase stability problems at elevated temperatures, as discussed in the Introduction.

The alumina thermal expansion data obtained in this study (Figure 6) compared compare relatively well with the literature values [21] from room temperature to 400°C. However, the thermal expansions measured in this study divergence from the literature values for temperatures greater than about 400°C

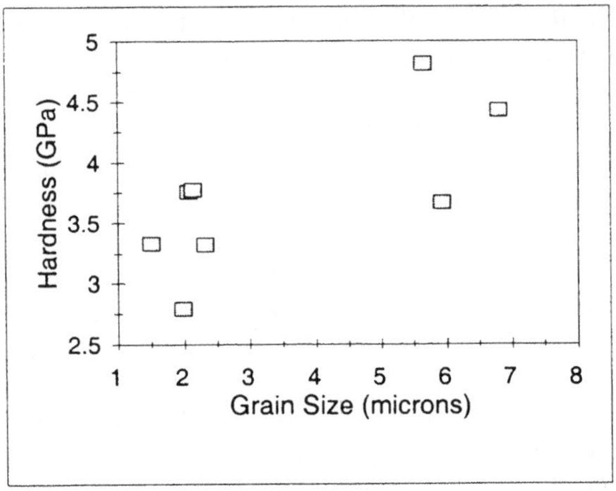

Figure 2 Hardness versus grain size for sintered hydroxyapatite

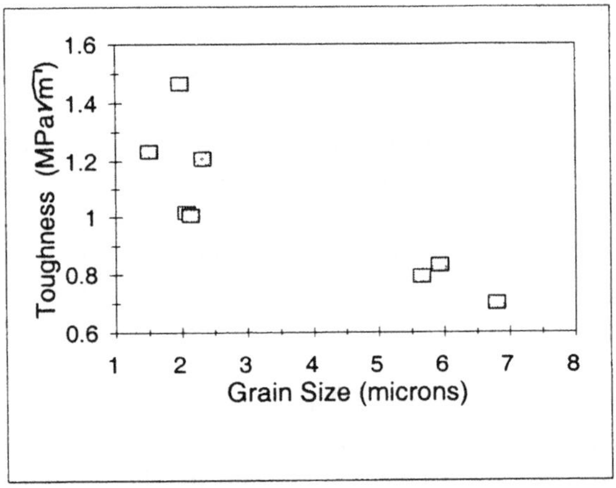

Figure 3 Toughness versus grain size for sintered hydroxyapatite

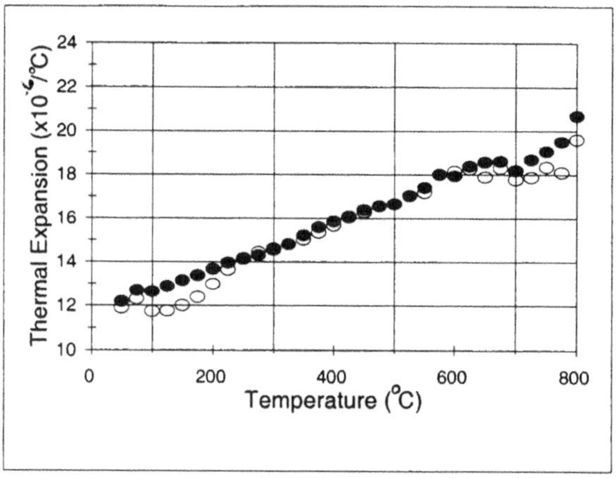

Figure 4 Smoothed thermal expansion data for sintered HAP specimens 4 (filled circles) and 12 (open circles)

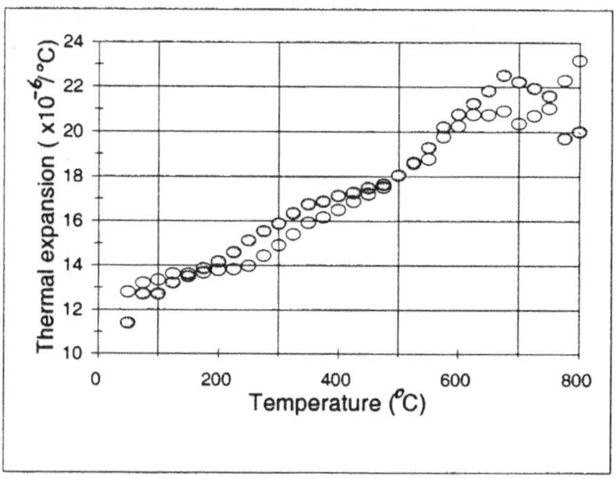

Figure 5 Smoothed thermal expansion data for sintered HAP specimens 5 (filled circles) and 11 (open circles)

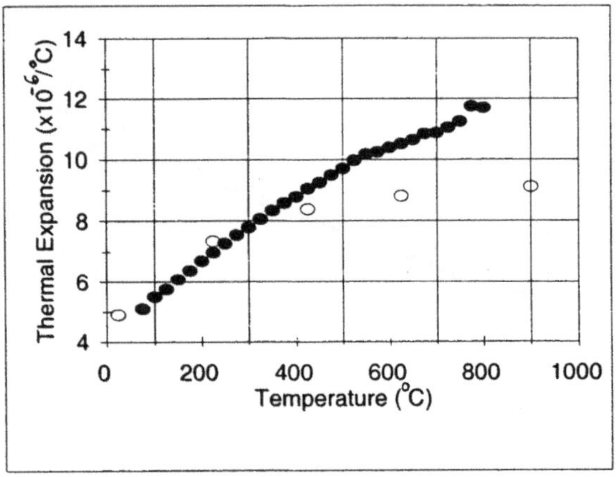

Figure 6 Averaged and smoothed thermal expansion data for sintered alumina (filled circles, this study) compared to alumina thermal expansion data from[22] (open circles)

(Figure 6). The alumina thermal expansion data (Figure 6) represents the average of a total of four thermal expansion trials.

CONCLUSIONS

Commercially available hydroxyapatite powders were sintered to a theoretical density of greater than 90% without significant phase decomposition. The average grain sizes in the sintered material were greater than 1.5 microns (Tables 1 and 2).

The fracture toughness and hardness data is consistent with microcracking in HAP, if critical grain size for HAP exceeds the smallest grain size (1.5 microns) included in this study. Microcracking likely exists in HAP due to the known thermal expansion anisotropy of HAP, as reviewed in the Introduction and Background sections of this paper. To produce HAP specimens whose fracture toughness and hardness are not functions of grain size [1], one would likely need to fabricate specimens with mean grain sizes smaller than the critical grain size, g_{cr}. Thus, the results of this study imply that the critical grain size is smaller than 1.5 microns, but further work is needed to better define the critical grain size for HAP.

REFERENCES

1. E. D. Case, J. R. Smyth, O. Hunter, Jr., "Microcrack Healing During Temperature Cycling of Single Phase Ceramics", *Fracture Mechanics of Ceramics, Volume 5*, Plenum Press (1983).
2. J. C. Elliott, *Structure and Chemistry of the Apatites and Other Calcium Orthophosphates*, Elsevier, (1994).
3. H. B. Van Rees, M. Mengot and E. Kostiner, "Monoclinic-Hexagonal Transition in Hydroxyapatite and Deuterohydroxyapatite Single Crystals", *Material Research Bulletin*, 8: 1307-1309, (1973).
4. G. R. Fischer, P. Bardhan, J. E. Geiger, "The lattice thermal expansion of hydroxyapatite", *Journal of Material Science Letters*, 2: 577-578 (1983).
5. W. G. Perdok, J. Christofferson, J. Arends, "The Thermal Lattice Expansion of Calcium Hydroxyapatite", *Journal of Crystal Growth*, 80: 149-154 (1987).
6. A. Royer, J. C. Viguie, M. Heughebaert, J. C. Heughebaert, "Stoichiometry of hydroxyapatite; influence on the flexural strength", *Journal of Materials Science: Materials in Medicine*, 4: 76-82 (1993).
7. P. E. Wang and T. K. Chaki, "Sintering behaviour and mechanical properties of hydroxyapatite and dicalcium phosphate", *Journal of Materials Science*: Materials in Medicine, 4: 150-158 (1993).

8. K. Yamashita, K. Kitagaki, and T. Umegaki, "Thermal Instability and Proton Conductivity of Ceramic Hydroxyapatite at High Temperatures", *Journal of the American Ceramic Society*, 78 [5]: 1191-1197 (1995).
9. Y. Fang, D. K. Agrawal, D. M. Roy, and R. Roy, "Microwave sintering of hydroxyapatite ceramics", *Journal of Material Research*, 9: 180-187 (1994).
10. W. L. Suchanek and M. Yoshimura, "Preparation of Fibrous, Porous Hydroxyapatite Ceramics from Hydroxyapatite Whiskers", *Journal of the American Ceramic Society*, 81: 765-767 (1998).
11. D. P. H. Hasselman, K. Y. Donaldson, E. M. Anderson and T. A. Johnson, "Effect of Thermal History on the Thermal Diffusivity and Thermal Expansion of an Alumina-Aluminum Titanate Composite", *Journal of the American Ceramic Society*, 76 [9]: 2180-2184 (1993).
12. T. Kijima and M. Tsutsumi, "Preparation and Thermal Properties of Dense Polycrystalline Oxyhydroxyapatite", *Journal of the American Ceramic Society*, 62 [9]: 455-460 (1979).
13. R.Halouani, D. Bernache-Assolant, E. Champion, A. Ababou, "Microstructure and related mechanical properties of hot pressed hydroxyapatite ceramics", *Journal of Materials Science: Materials in Medicine*, 5: 563-568 (1994)
14. J. J. Cleveland and R. C. Bradt, "Grain Size/Microcracking Relations for Pseudobrookite Oxides", *Journal of the American Ceramic Society*, 61: 478-481 (1978).
15. J. B. Wachtman, pp 82-84 in *Mechanical Properties of Ceramics*, John Wiley and Sons, New York, (1996).
16. W. L. Suchanek, M. Yashima, M. Kakihana and M. Yoshimura, "Hydroxyapatite/Hydroxyapatite-Whisker Composites without Sintering Additives: Mechanical Properties and Microstructural Evolution", *Journal of the American Ceramic Society*, 80[11]: 2805-2813 (1997).
17. R. W. Rice, C. C. Wu, and F. Borchelt, "Hardness -grain size relations in ceramics", *Journal of the American Ceramic Society*, 77: 2539-2553 (1994).
18. A. Knell and P. Blank, "Grain Size Dependence of Hardness in Dense Sub-micrometer Alumina", *J. Amer. Ceram. Soc.* 78: 1118-1120 (1995).
19. J. Ricote, L. Pardo, and B. Jiminez, "Mechanical characterization of calcium-modified lead titanate ceramics by indentation methods", *Journal of Materials Science* 29: 3248-3254 (1994).
20. R. W. Rice, "Grain size and porosity dependence of ceramic fracture energy and toughness at 22 C", *Journal of Materials Science* 31: 1969-1983 (1996).
21. *American Institute of Physics Handbook*, p. 4-72, Second Edition, McGraw-Hill Book Company, Inc., New York, NY, (1963).

SPRAY DRIED TITANIA CELL CARRIERS

K.-L. Eckert and E. Wintermantel
Biocompatible Materials Science and Engineering, ETH Zurich, Wagistrasse 23, CH-8952 Schlieren, Switzerland

R. Gadow
Institute for Manufacturing Technologies of Ceramic Components and Composites, University of Stuttgart, Allmandring 5b, D-70569 Stuttgart, Germany

ABSTRACT

Hollow alumina and titania granulates were developed which could be used as cell carriers for biomedical applications. The influence of slurry properties, binder content and solids content on the formation of hollow granulates was investigated. The slurries were characterized by density and rheological measurements using oscillation rheometry. Granulate size distributions were determined by laser diffraction after sintering. Granulate morphology was investigated by SEM. The investigations showed that hollow granulates with suitable geometries can be produced with optimized parameters. The influence of binder additions was lower than the effects of slurry rheology and solids contents. The tap densities and mean granulate sizes decreased with lower solids content. For producing hollow granulates an optimum range of solids contents exists both for alumina and titania.

INTRODUCTION

Polycrystalline ceramics such as alumina or titania are highly hydrophilic and chemically stable in physiological media. Therefore these types of ceramic materials can serve as substrate materials for cell culture in biomedical applications and as implants. Titania ceramics have been demonstrated to be a favorable substrate material for liver cell culture [1]. For cell transplantation, hollow granulates with an opening have been found to be favorable, in order to support blood vessel ingrowth into the internal cavity and enabling a complex and physiological vascular supply for cells transplanted on the carrier [2, 3]. In former work hollow granulates have been produced from alumina slurries by forming drops of slurry on a heated surface [4]. Spray drying could be an alternative shaping method enabling to produce large numbers of hollow spheres. The goal of this work was to develop spray-dried hollow particles with spherical shape in a size range of 100-200 µm. The internal volume of the particles should be as large as possible to minimize the ceramic bulk content and thereby the amounts of synthetic materials used in cell culturing or cell transplantation.

The formation of hollow granulates during spray drying has been attributed to four mechanisms [5]: occurrence of a semipermeable membrane at the surface of a droplet; precipitation of soluble compounds at the droplet surface; pore formation due to air bubbles in the slurry; transport of insoluble solids to the droplet periphery. The formation of a void space within a droplet creates a vacuum which leads to collapsing or imploding. Thus hollow particles are formed with an opening which makes the void space accessible from the outside.

The production of hollow granulates has been investigated for refractory applications [6], for polishing media [7], and for adsorption media in chromatography [8]. All authors concluded that slurry viscosity had a major influence on the formation of hollow granulates. This included deflocculation as well as solids content in the slurries investigated. Complete deflocculation was reported to be essential as well as not too high a solids content in the slurry. The influence of organic additives was investigated by [9] indicating that formation of organic membranes at the droplet periphery can also be an important factor for void space formation during spray drying.

In this work the formation of hollow particles during spray drying of alumina and titania slurries was investigated. Binder content and solids content were varied. The viscosity of the slurries was measured and the spray-dried powders prepared were analyzed determining granulate size distribution, tap density and granulate morphology.

MATERIALS AND METHODS

Alumina

A standard slurry was prepared from alumina powders, deflocculator and demineralized water. The grain size distribution of the homogenized slurry is displayed in table I. This slurry was then supplemented with binders and additional water to adjust solids contents. The slurries were stirred for 24 h and sieved at 125 µm prior to spraying.

Two experimental series were performed, one for investigation of binder additions and one to investigate the effect of solids content. For the first series the basic slurry was supplemented with 0.7, 1.0 and 2.2 % polycarbonate binder and diluted to a solids content of 73.2 %. For the second series the slurry was diluted to solids contents of 83.2, 73.2, 70.6, 68.2 and 63.8 %. In this series the binder content was 1.5 % of the solids content in the respective slurry.

Titania

A standard slurry with 65.4 % solids content was prepared from titania powder (specific surface area 8.3 m^2g^{-1}), deflocculator, binder and demineralized water. The grain size distribution of the homogenized slurry is displayed in table I. This slurry was then supplemented with additional water to adjust solids contents to 59.6 and 46.5 %. The slurries were stirred for 24 h and sieved at 125 µm prior to spraying. In a second experimental run slurries with 39.7, 48.7 and 62.0 wt% solids content were prepared, corresponding to 10, 20 and 30 vol% solids content. Binder and deflocculator additions were adapted at each step to minimize the changes in viscosity which were caused by the different solids contents.

Spray drying

A mixed flow spray dryer (Nubilosa) with 18 kW power output and about 5 kg/h water evaporation capacity was used. For atomization, a two-fluid nozzle with 1.2 mm orifice operated at 75 kPa air pressure was applied. Inlet air temperature was 225° C. Outlet temperature was kept at 90-110° C by controlling the slurry flow rate which ranged from 1.0-2.0 l/h depending on the solids content. The slurries were stirred to prevent sedimentation of solids. The resulting product was filled into alumina crucibles and sintered at 1550° C (alumina) or 1150° C (titania) applying a heating rate of 3 K/min and a holding time of 25 min. Deagglomeration after sintering was performed manually by pestle and mortar.

Characterization

Grain size distributions of the slurries was measured by laser diffraction (Mastersizer S, Malvern), specific surface was determined by nitrogen adsorption. Viscous properties were measured with a rheometer (UDS 200, Physica), in the oscillating mode at 1 Hz using a plate-plate setup with 1.0 mm gap width and in a shear stress range of 0-100 Pa.

The sintered granulates were sieved using sieves with 140 µm and 100 µm mesh width. Tap density of each of the above mentioned fractions was determined by filling a calibrated 1.2 ml-pipette with granulate and vibrating by light tapping until no further compaction was observed. The reproducibility of the volume measurement was determined to be better than ±0.01 ml. To compare tap densities of alumina and titania, obtained values were calculated as fractions of the respective true densities of 3.965 g/cm^3 for alumina and 4.26 g/cm^3 for titania (rutile).

Grain size distributions of the slurries, of as-sprayed materials and of sieved fractions were measured by laser diffraction (Malvern). Granulate morphology was investigated by scanning electron microscopy (SEM, Hitachi).

RESULTS

Slurry properties

The mean grain size of the alumina slurry is greater than that of the titania slurry (table I). Rheological measurements showed that for both alumina and titania the loss modulus was by orders of magnitude greater than the storage modulus (figure 2). Thus, the rheological behavior was controlled by viscosity and not by elastic effects. It was therefore possible to take the amount of the complex viscosity $|\eta^*|$ for characterizing the rheological behavior

Alumina, At high solids contents in the slurries shear thinning could be observed in the low-shear range and weak dilatancy at high shear. The more diluted slurries < 40 vol% solids content showed Newtonian behavior in the investigated shear stress range (figure 1). In these slurries sedimentation of the solid compound occurred. At intermediate and high shear stresses, the viscosities of alumina slurries were similar for all investigated compositions (figure 4). The binder addition had its greatest influence at low shear stress (1 Pa). At higher shear stresses, viscosity behavior was not affected by the shear stress as can be seen from the similarity of the viscosity values measured at 20 and 40 Pa (figure 2).

Titania, The viscosities of titania slurries were in the same order of magnitude as the alumina slurries, but showed a stronger dependence from the solids content (figure 4). Shear thinning in the low shear range and dilatancy at high shear were more pronounced than with alumina slurries (figure 3) Newtonian behavior was observed for slurries containing less than 20 vol% of titania powder.

Table I: Grain size distributions

	Alumina slurries	Titania slurries
D_{10} (μm)	0.48	0.30
D_{50} (μm)	2.55	0.74
D_{90} (μm)	9.45	1.92

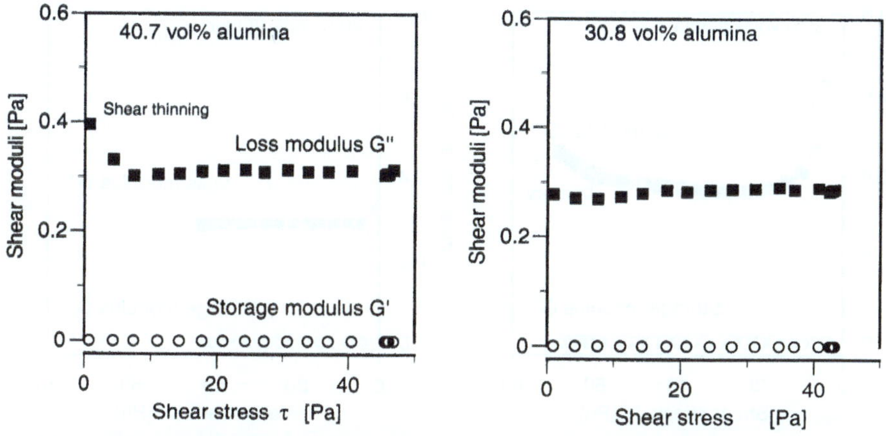

Figure 1: Oscillating viscosity measurements of alumina slurries. Left: slurry with 73.2 % solids, right: slurry with 68.2 % solids.

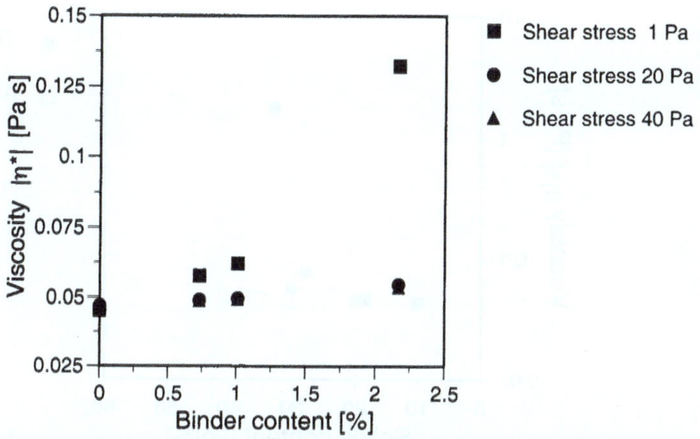

Figure 2: Viscosity data for alumina slurries containing different amounts of binder, measured at different shear stress levels. All slurries had 73.2 % solids content.

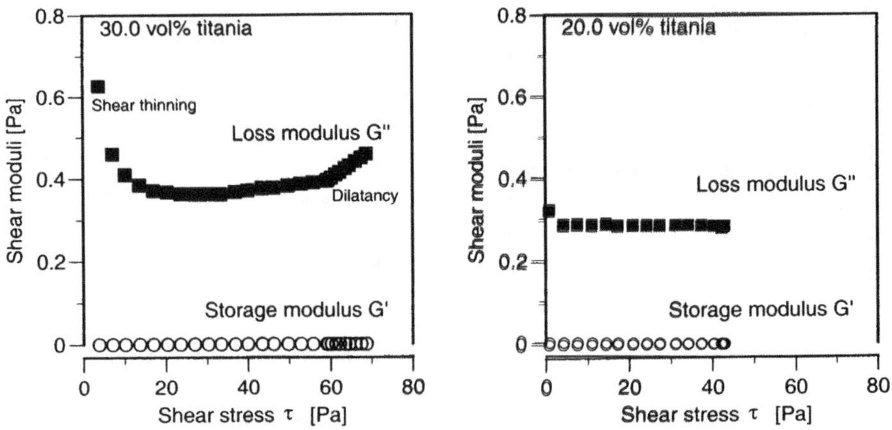

Figure 3: Oscillating viscosity measurements of titania slurries. Left: slurry with 62.0 % solids, right: slurry with 48.7 % solids.

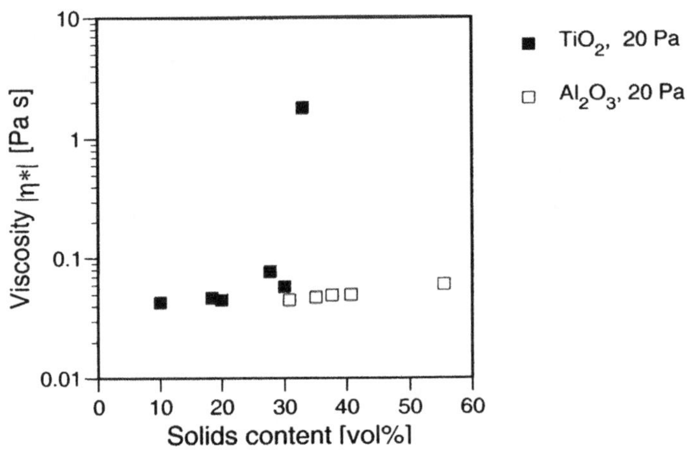

Figure 4: Viscosities of titania and alumina slurries as function of the volume fraction of solids in the slurry, measured at 20 Pa shear stress.

Alumina granulate properties

Binder additions and changes in solids contents on the slurries had only small effects on the mean grain sizes of the granulates (figure 5). The tap densities measured for the alumina granulate depended on the size of the fraction. The highest tap densities were measured for the fraction < 100 µm, whereas the fraction > 140 m exhibited the lowest tap densities in all samples investigated. Binder additions to the slurry did not have a clear effect. The tap densities did not change systematically for a range of binder additions (figure 6). The values were at a constant level. On the other hand, the solids content in the slurry affected the tap densities clearly. Increasing tap densities were measured with increasing solids contents; in particular for the fractions >140 µm and 100-140 µm. The tap densities appear to be linearly correlated with the solids contents of the slurries. (figure 7). Morphological investigation by SEM showed that most granulates were hollow. The internal cavities were found to be partly filled with small granulates (figure 8). Investigation of the dimensions of the internal cavities revealed that the internal cavities were not larger in size than 50 % of the granulate diameter (figure 9).

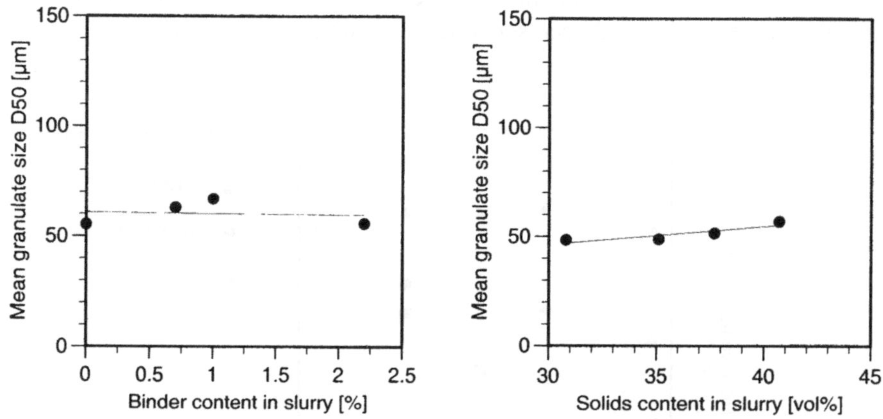

Figure 5: Left: Development of granulate size distribution sprayed from alumina slurries with different binder contents. Right: Granulate size distribution measured after spraying slurries with different solids contents.

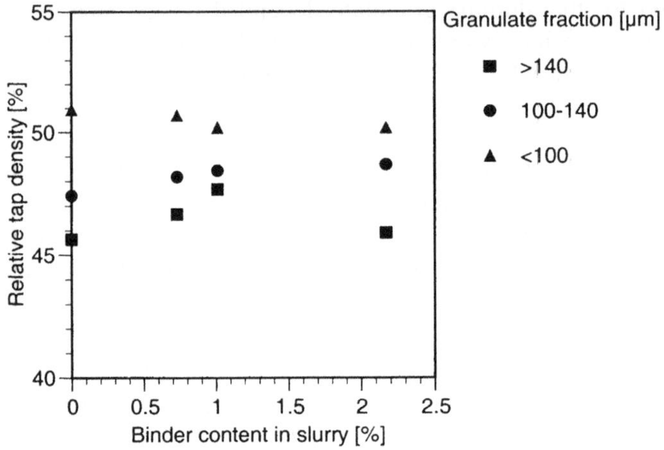

Figure 6: Influence of binder content on the relative tap density of spray-dried alumina granulates which had been separated into different fractions.

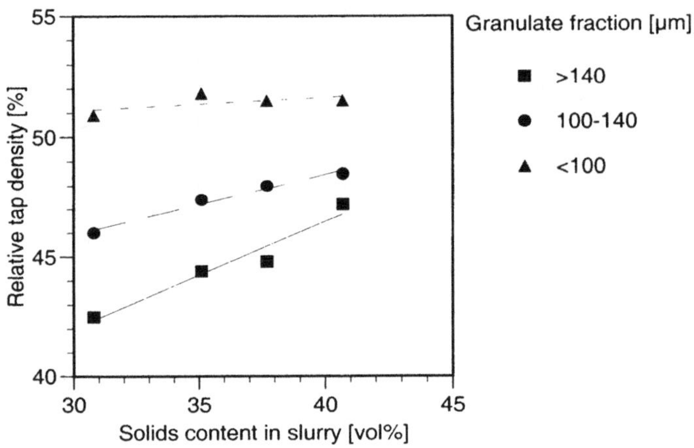

Figure 7: Relative tap densities of alumina granulate fractions >140 µm, 100-140 µm and <100 µm as function of the solids content in the slurry.

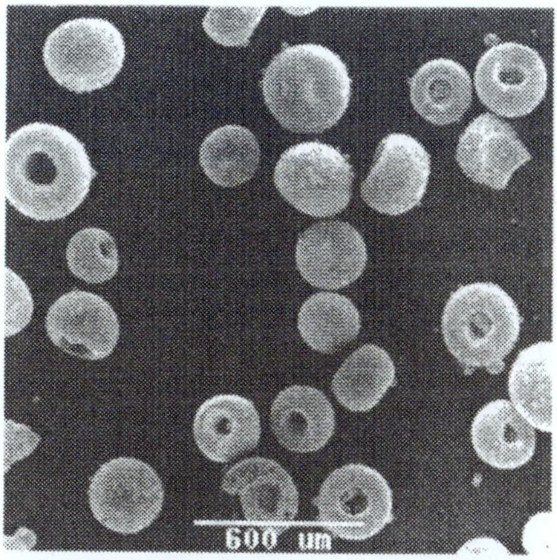

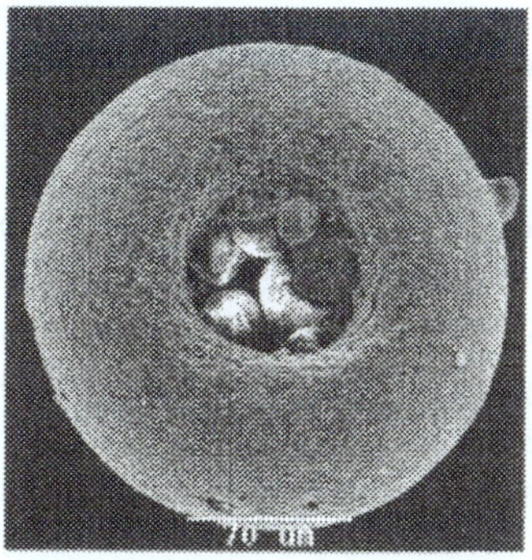

Figure 8: Morphology of spray-dried alumina granulates, sieved fraction > 140 μm. These granulates were sprayed with a solids content of 73.2% (left). Right: view of a single granulate.

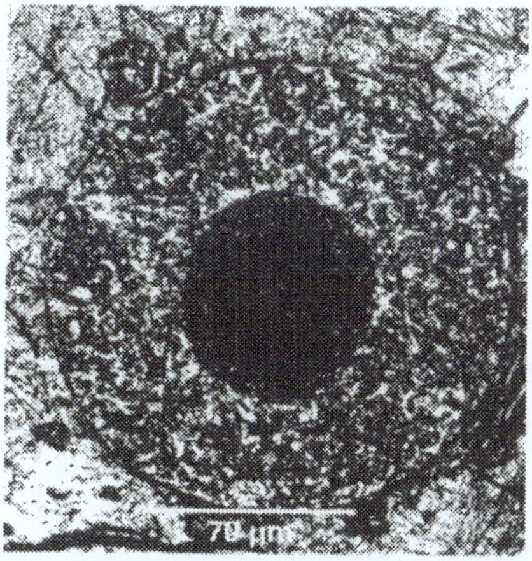

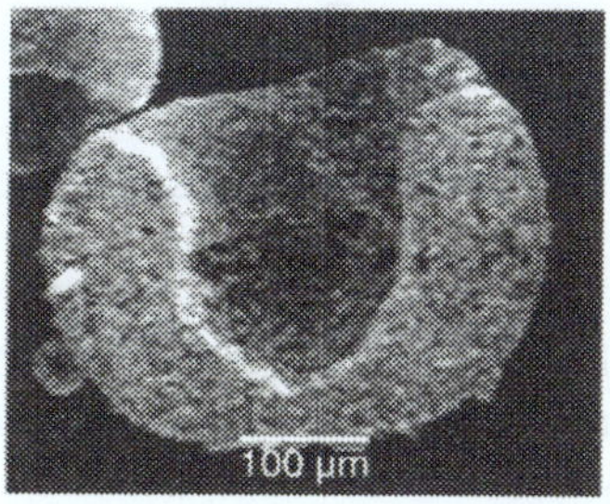

Figure 9: Sections through alumina granulates (> 140 μm) showing the relation between external and internal diameter. Left: CLSM-image of a ground section. Right: Side view (SEM).

Titania granulate properties

The mean size D_{50} of the as-sprayed granulates increased with increasing solids content in the slurry (figure 10). This effect was stronger than with alumina. Similarly, the tap densities increased with higher solids contents (figure 11). The granulate morphology observed by SEM reflects the behavior of the tap density. The morphology of the granulates remained constant for intermediate and high solids contents, an increase in opening diameter was observed with decreasing solids content (figure 12). At solids contents below 45 % the particle morphology tended to be irregular, with small particles adhering to the large ones (figure 13). Large granules obtained from these slurries had internal cavities greater than those obtained from slurries with higher solids contents, but often displayed oval shapes (figure 12).

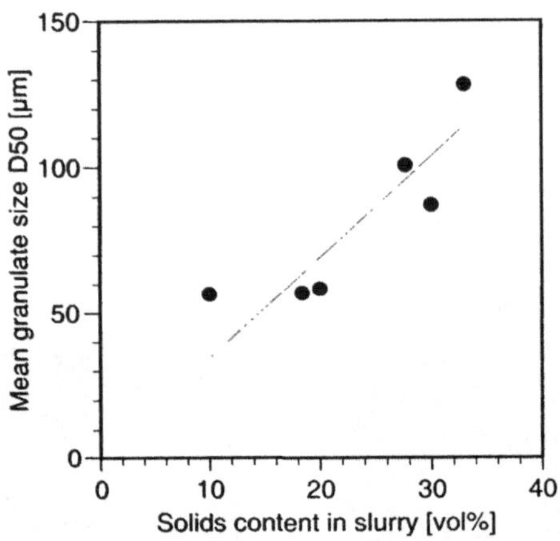

Figure 10: Granulate size of titania granulates as function of the solids content in the slurry. The mean particle size of the as-sprayed titania granulates increases strongly with the solid content.

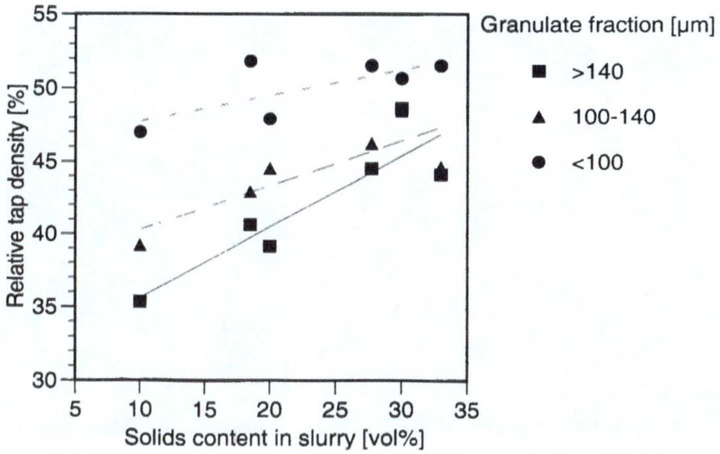

Figure 11: Relative tap density as function of the solid contents in the slurries. The tap densities of all fractions are affected by the increasing solids content. The smaller fractions exhibit higher tap densities

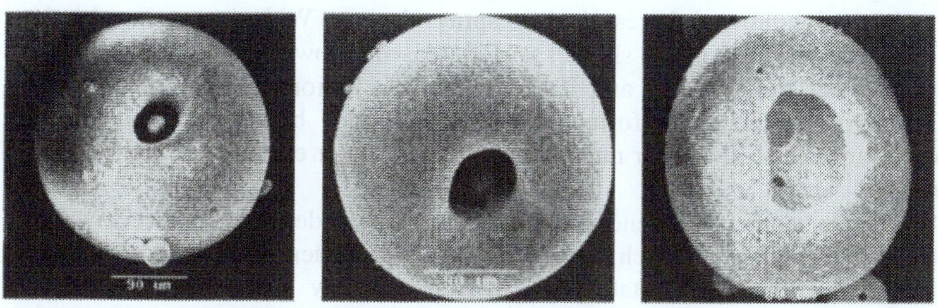

Figure 12: Morphology of hollow titania granulates, made from a slurries containing 64.5 % solid (left), 59.6 vol% solid (middle) and 46.5 % solid (right).

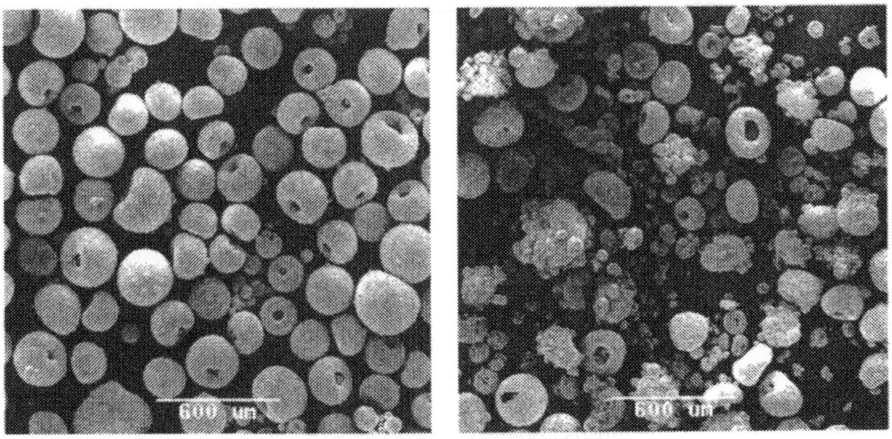

Figure 13: Morphology of titania granulates sprayed from slurries with high and intermediate solids contents (left) and sprayed from slurries with low solids contents (right)

DISCUSSION

The goal of this work was to investigate the role of slurry properties in the formation of hollow spheres during spray drying. With increasing binder additions the viscosity of the slurries was increased at low shear stresses whereas at higher shear stresses of 20 and 40 Pa the binder additions had only little effect. This behavior reflects the formation of weak bonds between the individual powder particles at low shear rates, which are no longer effective at higher shear rates.

The binder content influenced particle size and tap density only weakly. The pseudoplastic behavior which can be created by binder addition can thus be utilized to prevent sedimentation in slurries with low solids content without affecting morphological particle properties such as size and shape.

The beneficial effects of reduced solids content in slurries for production of hollow granulates, which have been reported by other authors [6-8] could be confirmed by the results of this work. The tap densities of alumina and of titania granulates appeared to be linearly correlated with the solids content in the slurry, indicating that a defined correlation may exist between solids content and shape of the granulates.

The particle size distribution after spray drying was also positively correlated with the solids content in the slurry. This means for the production of large granulates, that on the one hand high solids content is favorable for the formation of the large granulates which are desired for application as cell carriers. On the other hand this leads to high tap densities, i.e. granulates with a small internal volume.

The development of a hollow shape is also influenced by the relation between heat and mass transfer during the drying process. These two aspects will be the objectives of further optimization.

CONCLUSIONS AND OUTLOOK

Size distribution and the formation of hollow granulates during spray drying were more strongly influenced by the solids content in the slurry than by binder additions. Both types of materials tested, alumina and titania, showed similar behaviors. It can be concluded that the yield of hollow granulates of the desired size range of 100-200 μm can be optimized by adapting the solids content in the slurries. The shape of the granulates is similar to the shape of those cell carriers which have been produced by dropping slurry on a hot surface [1]. Further morphological investigations are necessary to investigate the internal structure and the surface-to-volume ratio of the developed granulates.

ACKNOWLEDGEMENTS

The authors would like to acknowledge the fruitful discussions and laboratory assistance of A. Corzilius R. Fischer, M. Lischka and G. Schäfer, Institute for Manufacturing Technologies of Ceramic Components and Composites, University of Stuttgart.

REFERENCES

[1] K.-L. Eckert, B. Stieger, R. Meier-Abt, R. Gadow and E. Wintermantel, "*Titania ceramic surfaces as scaffolds for hepatocyte culture*", Proceedings of the International Conference on Engineering Ceramics and Structures, Larry Hench Symposium on Surface-Active Processes in Materials, Cocoa Beach, U.S.A., 1999, in press.

[2] K.-L. Eckert, P. Groscurth, R. Gadow and E. Wintermantel, "*Implantable ceramic cell carriers for liver cell transplantation*", Proceedings of the 6. Interregional European Ceramics Colloquium "Advanced Ceramics and Composites" (IEKC 6), Stuttgart, Germany, 1998, in press.

[3] E. Wintermantel, L. Cima, B. Schloo and R. Langer, "Angiopolarity of cell carriers: directional angiogenesis in resorbable liver cell transplantation devices"; pp. 331-334 in *Angiogenesis: Key Principles-Science-Technology-Medicine*, edited by R. Steiner, P. B. Weisz and R. Langer. Birkhaeuser Verlag Basel, Switzerland, 1992.

[4] K.-L. Eckert, U. Rösler, M. Mathey, J. Mayer, E. Wintermantel and H. Hofmann, "Open porous ceramics for cell transplantation devices: a new biomaterial - first results"; pp. 251-255 in *Bioceramics 6*, edited by P. Ducheyne and D. Christiansen. Butterworth-Heinemann Ltd. Oxford, UK, 1993.

[5] S.J. Lukasiewicz, "Spray-drying ceramic powders", *J. Am. Ceram. Soc.*, 72 617-624 (1989).

[6] H.J. Eitel, "Entwicklung und Produktion von Giesspulvergranulat mittels Sprühtrocknungsverfahren sowie dessen Bedeutung für die Stahlindustrie (Development and production of granulated casting powder using spray drying technology and its significance for the steel industry)", Ph.D.-Thesis, Rheinisch-Westfälische Technische Hochschule, Aachen, Germany, 1990

[7] N.B. Kirk and J.V. Wood, "The effect of the calcination process on the crystallite shape of sol-gel cerium oxide used for glass polishing", *J. Mater. Sci.*, 30 2171-2175 (1995).

[8] P. Luo and T.G. Nieh, "Preparing hydroxyapatite powders with controlled morphology", *Biomaterials*, 17 1959-1964 (1996).

[9] Büttiker, "Erzeugung von gleich grossen Tropfen mit suspendiertem und geloestem Feststoff und deren Trocknung im freien Fall (Generation of equisized drops containing suspended or dissolved solids and their drying in free fall)", Ph.D.-Thesis, Eidgenössische Technische Hochschule, Zurich, Switzerland, 1978

CRYSTALLIZATION OF SIC ON BIOLOGICAL CARBON PRECOURSERS

H. Sieber*, H. Friedrich, A.Kaindl and P.Greil,

University of Erlangen-Nuremberg, Department of Materials Science (III), Glass and Ceramics, D-91058 Erlangen, Germany

ABSTRACT

The reaction kinetics and crystallization behavior of β-SiC on Si-coated cellulose fibres and in Si-infiltrated carbon preforms derived from wood structures was investigated. After heat treatment at a temperature of 1450°C the cellulose fibers were completely transformed into β-SiC. Depending on the infiltration process (liquid or gaseous) different SiC morphologies were formed. The β-SiC grains formed inside the porous wood structure by liquid Si infiltration were found to exhibit a microcrystalline texture indicating a preferred crystallographic orientation of the β-SiC particles. The texture can be explained by the transformation of the initial microfibrils in the cell wall of the wood into highly ordered carbon fibrils during pyrolysis and an oriented nucleation ($(110)_{SiC} \parallel (0001)_C$) of the SiC particles after Si infiltration. The kinetics of the reaction processes will be discussed and compared with the formation of SiC particles on synthetic carbon substrates.

1. INTRODUCTION

Biological composite materials developed from nature in a long-term genetic evolution process often show superior structure-mechanical property relationships in comparison to synthetic materials. Due to their hierarchically built structural morphology, materials like wood and natural fibre composites exhibit an excellent strength at low density, high stiffness and elasticity, and damage tolerance on a micro as well as on a macro scale [1-5]. The mechanical properties of wood like materials are determined by the open cellular structure and an uniaxial pore morphology resulting in a pronounced anisotropy of the elasticity, deformation and fracture behavior. Various micro mechanical models were derived to describe the mechanical properties of cellular materials with different porosity [6-8].

Conversion of biological structures into inorganic (ceramic) materials has attained particular interest [9-12]. Biological structures can be used as template structures such as carbonized wood to process materials with definite porosity on the micrometer scale, or the materials can be easily preprocessed in forms of natural fibres, husk or shells (see Table 1). In natural plant structures, the syntheses rate can be significantly increased by using the internal open porosity system for gaseous or liquid infiltration.

Table 1: Processing of biological structures into ceramic materials.

TEMPLATE	PROCESS	PRODUCT
Wood structures:	Infiltration of the raw or dried porous wood with metal-organic suspension like TEOS (tetraethyl orthosilicate) and subsequent high-temperature pyrolysis [13].	SiC ceramics.
	Pyrolysis of dried wood to obtain carbon preforms. Infiltration and reaction with liquid or gaseous Si [14].	SiC or SiSiC ceramics.
Natural fibres:	Infiltration of sisal, jute and hamp fibres with $AlCl_3$ and $TiCl_4$, respectively, and subsequently annealing in air [15, 16].	Oxidic Al_2O_3 and TiO_2 fibres.
	Cotton fibres coated with Si_3N_4 and subsequent annealing in Ar-atmosphere at 1200-1600°C [17].	SiC fibres.
Rice husk:	Pyrolysis of dried rice husk in N_2-atmosphere at 1400°C ([18]).	SiC whiskers.
Coconut shells:	Pyrolysis of crushed pieces of dried coconut shells in Ar-atmosphere at 1400°C [19].	SiC whiskers.

In the present paper, the reaction kinetics and phase nucleation of SiC were investigated on carbonized biological preforms derived from cellulose fibres and natural wood. Paper composed of pure cellulose fibres and wood of different pore size distribution were carbonized at different temperatures. Subsequently the carbon templates e.g. fibres or carbonized wood were coating with Si and converted into β-SiC. Different SiC morphologies were formed on the fibres and the wood templates. The β-SiC reaction kinetics, phase morphology and crystal orientations will be related to the processing parameters, the morphology of the carbonized biomaterials and the initial cellulose microfibril orientation in the natural grown wood.

2. EXPERIMENTAL PROCEDURE

Paper consisting of pure cellulose fibres (cleaning and filter paper, Whatman, Hardened Ashless Grade 540:8μm) and various kinds of natural wood (oak, beech, pine, ebony, maple, balsa) with different fractional densities and porosity structures were used as biological templates for conversion into SiC-ceramics. The papers were pyrolyzed in argon atmosphere at a temperature of 1400°C for 4 hs. The wood specimens were dried and subsequently pyrolyzed in N_2-atmosphere in a carbon heated furnace at a temperature of up to 1800°C for 4 hs. During pyrolysis a slow heating rate of 1°C/min was applied up to 500°C where the polyaromatic hydrocarbon polymers (cellulose, hemicellulose, lignin) have completely decomposed to carbon followed by a higher rate of 5°C/min up to the peak temperature.

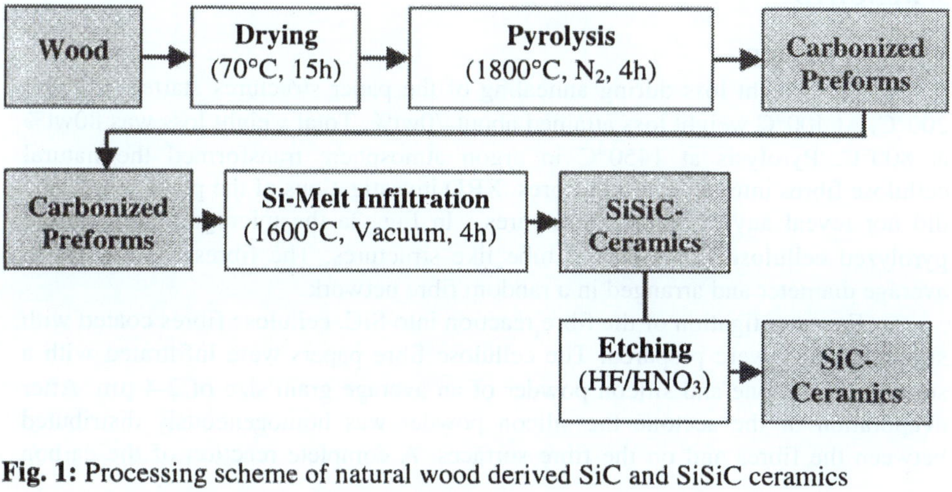

Fig. 1: Processing scheme of natural wood derived SiC and SiSiC ceramics

The porous carbon preforms were infiltrated with liquid silicon in carbon dies at 1600°C without pressure according to the conventional processing of SiSiC-materials [20-22]. The specimens were kept for 4 hs at this temperature to allow complete reaction of silicon with the carbon structure to form β-SiC. Unreacted silicon remained in part of the pore channels so that a cellular Si-containing SiC composite material finally was obtained. For investigation of the orientation of the formed β-SiC grains, the residual silicon was etched in an aqueous solution of HF/HNO_3 at room temperature. The processing scheme is summarized in Fig. 1.

The organic → inorganic conversion of the biological material was monitored by thermal balance analysis (TGA, STA 409, Netzsch Gerätebau, Selb, Germany). Density and porosity were measured by Helium pycnometry (Accu Pyk 1330, Micromeritics, Düsseldorf, Germany). Distribution of tracheidal cell diameters was determined by stereological analysis of SEM micrographs of axial cross sections. The microstructures of the intermediate and final products were characterized by scanning electron microscopy (SEM, Stereoscan S 250 MK3, Cambridge Instruments, Cambridge, UK) and elemental analysis by EDX/SEM and WDX/SEM. The crystalline phases were determined by X-ray diffraction using CuK_{α} radiation (XRD, D 500, Siemens, Karlsruhe, Germany). Electron backscattered analysis with 20 kV (EBSD, Link Oxford, Oxford, GB) was used to identify preferential orientations of ß-SiC formed by the solid-liquid reaction of silicon with the carbon preform.

3. RESULTS

3.1 CELLULOSE

The weight loss during annealing of the paper structures started at about 200°C. At 400°C weight loss attained about 70wt%. Total weight loss was 80wt% at 800°C. Pyrolysis at 1450°C in argon atmosphere transformed the natural cellulose fibres into pure carbon fibres. XRD investigations of the pyrolyzed fibres did nor reveal any crystalline structures. In Fig. 2a the micrograph shows the pyrolyzed cellulose fibres as flat tube like structures. The fibres are 10 μm in average diameter and arranged in a random fibre network.

For investigation of the fibre reaction into SiC, cellulose fibres coated with silicon powder were prepared. The cellulose fibre papers were infiltrated with a solution of acetone and silicon powder of an average grain size of 2-4 μm. After evaporation of the acetone the silicon powder was homogeneously distributed between the fibres and on the fibre surfaces. A complete reaction of the carbon fibre into SiC was achieved with some residual molten Si grains still visible in the reacted structure (Fig. 2b).

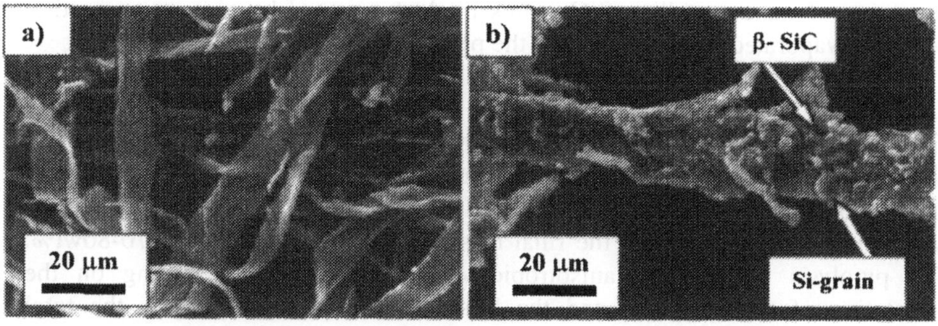

Fig. 2: a) SEM micrograph of the pyrolyzed cellulose fibre at 1450°C in argon, b) cellulose fibre coated with silicon.

As shown by XRD analysis, the crystallization of SiC started at a temperatures below 1200°C. After pyrolysis, the carbon content was analyzed by recording the weight loss during annealing in air. The TGA analysis did not show any residual carbon in the specimen after annealing at 1450°C. All the carbon of the cellulose fibres has been reacted into SiC ceramic.

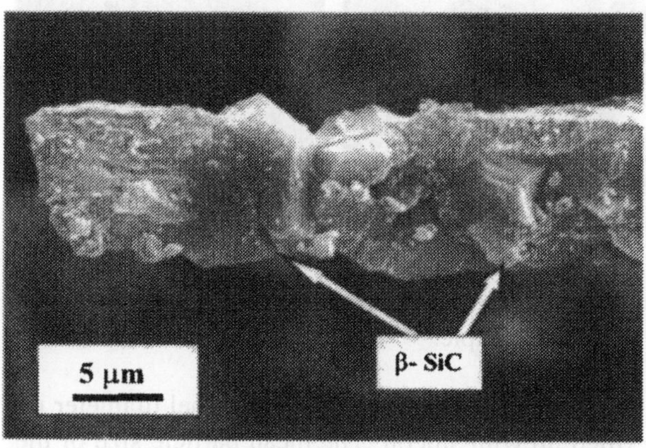

Fig. 3: SEM micrograph of a SiC fibre after reaction at 1450°C in argon atmosphere.

While large single crystalline SiC grains up to 10 μm in size were often observed close to unreacted silicon (see Fig. 2b, 3), long parts of the initial cellulose fibres seem to be without larger SiC grains and exhibit a fibre like morphology. The formation of nanocrystalline SiC grains might be caused by a gaseous reaction between evaporated Si and carbon on the porous fibre surface.

3.2 WOOD-COMPOSITE SYSTEM

The carbonized preforms exhibit a multimodal pore size distribution with pores between 1 to 200 μm. The weight loss during heating of the wood preforms is similar to the pure cellulose fibres. Due to the lignin content, which shows a weight loss of about 50wt%, the final loss of wood was found to be 70-80wt%. The pyrolysis involves an anisotropic shrinkage of 30% depending on the orientation of the specimen and the kind of wood. After pyrolysis the total porosity of carbonized wood is 20...25% higher than the initial density of (dried) wood [14]. Despite the changes in porosity and anisotropic shrinkage the porous macro- and microstructure of the carbonized wood is retained after pyrolysis with high precision, see Fig. 4.

When the carbonized wood preform was brought into contact with the silicon melt spontaneous wetting and infiltration of the porous structure occurred. XRD analysis proved that after infiltration with the silicon melt at 1600°C the carbon has completely transformed into the β-SiC phase.

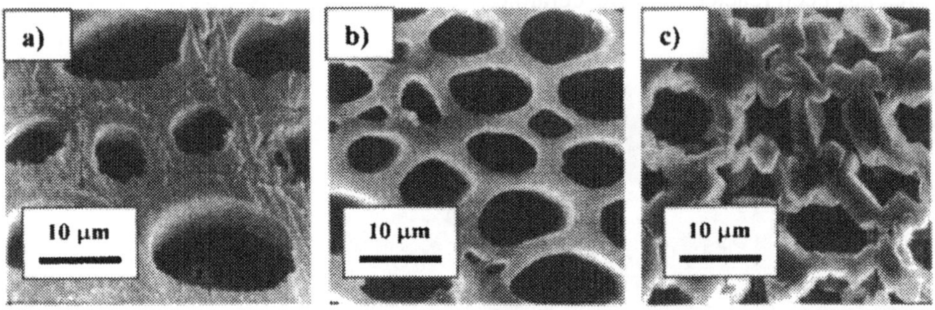

Fig. 4: SEM micrographs of a) natural grown, b) pyrolyzed (1800°C, 4h, N_2) and c) silicon infiltrated (1600°C, 4h, argon) maple.

After Si infiltration, pores in the infiltrated structure with an channel diameter up to approximately 30 μm were filled up with silicon. The mean particle size of the β-SiC grains is typically in the range of 5 μm.

Fig. 5 shows the EBSD patterns of ß-SiC-crystals surrounding a tracheidal pore channel on an axial plane (residual silicon has been etched out of the pore channel). Analysis of orientation symmetry of the (001), (110) and (100) diffraction patterns suggests the ß-SiC crystals are not randomly oriented but show a preferential crystallographic orientationship. The possibility of oriented nucleation of β-SiC with respect to the microscopic and mesoscopic structure of the pyrolyzed cellular carbon structure will be discussed later.

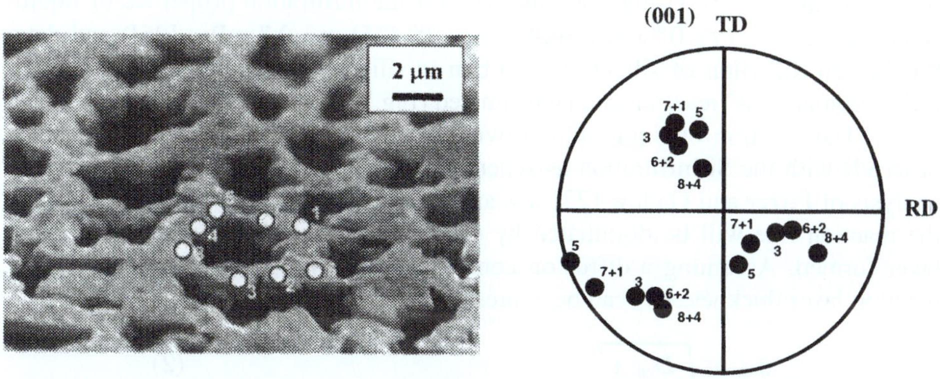

Fig. 5: EBSD pattern of β-SiC grains surrounding a tracheidal pore (Si was etched out by a HF/HNO_3 solution).

4. DISCUSSION

In the pure cellulose fibre specimens two different reaction morphologies of SiC were observed, that could be related to the contact of liquid silicon to the carbon fibre and thus to a liquid-solid or gaseous-solid reaction of the silicon with the carbon preform. Carbon fibre parts in contact with molten silicon exhibit the formation of large single SiC crystallites up to 10 µm in diameter. Carbon fibres not in direct contact with silicon were reacted into a nanocrystalline SiC ceramics exhibiting the shape of the original carbon fibre (Fig. 2b).

The SiC formation in the wood derived carbon preforms can be described as a $liquid_{Si}$-$solid_{carbon}$ reaction process. Spontaneous wetting of the silicon melt on the carbonized wood results in a very fast infiltration of the tracheidal pore channel system of the porous carbon preforms and concurrent reaction to form ß-SiC. For conversion of the bulk carbonized wood into SiC ceramics, the times required to achieve complete silicon infiltration of the porous carbon structure and to achieve complete reaction to the SiC phase are limited by the infiltration and reaction kinetics which are both functions of temperature.

The infiltration depth d_{inf} can be expressed as a function of time t by [20]:

$$d_{inf} \approx \sqrt{t\,[\frac{\gamma\, r \cos\Theta}{2\eta}]} \qquad (1)$$

and depends on the effective capillary geometry r and the properties of the infiltrating liquid e.g. surface tension γ, wetting angle Θ and viscosity η (see schematic in Fig. 6a). Using literature data for the infiltration properties of liquid silicon at 1600°C ($\gamma = 0.82$ N/m [24], $\Theta = 10°$ [25], $\eta = 0.7$ mPas [26]) and data for the self-diffusion of silicon and carbon in silicon carbide the time of silicon infiltration and SiC reaction can be estimated (Fig. 6b).

The reaction of liquid silicon with carbon to form ß-SiC simultaneously proceeds with the Si-infiltration as schematically indicated by Fig. 6a. A detailed analysis of Fitzer and Gadow [23] revealed that after complete wetting is reached the reaction rate will be dominated by diffusion through the primary solid SiC-layer formed. Assuming a diffusion controlled parabolic growth rate of SiC the reaction layer thickness d_{rea} can be expressed by:

$$d_{rea} = \sqrt{D_{eff}\ t} \qquad (2)$$

with $D_{eff} = D_0 \exp(-Q/RT)$ $\qquad Q = 132$ kJ/mol, $D_0 = 2 * 10^6$ cm/s

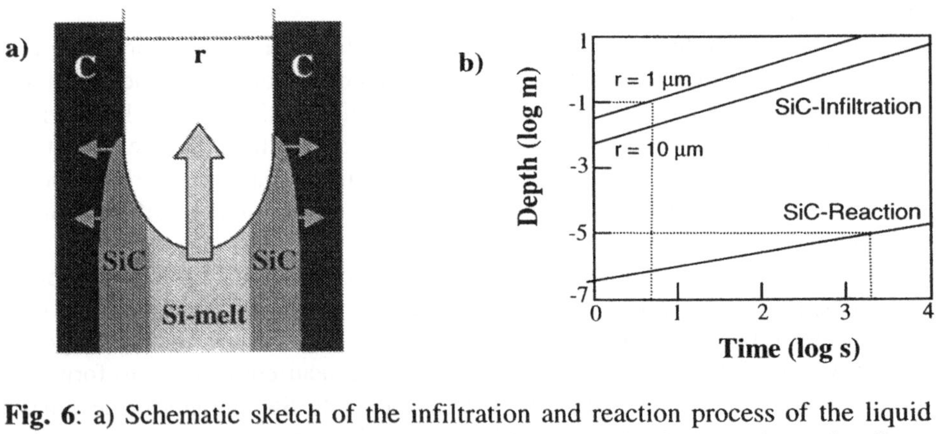

Fig. 6: a) Schematic sketch of the infiltration and reaction process of the liquid silicon into the porous carbon preform. b) Infiltration depth d_{inf} and reaction layer thickness d_{rea} at 1600°C calculated with equation (1) and (2).

The variation of infiltration depth and reaction layer thickness with time for a range of pore radii and cell wall thicknesses are shown in Fig. 6b. The ratio of infiltration depth to reaction layer thickness:

$$d_{inf} / d_{rea} \quad > \quad 10^5 \qquad (4)$$

indicates that the SiC reaction rate is the rate controlling factor in the overall wood-ceramic conversion process.

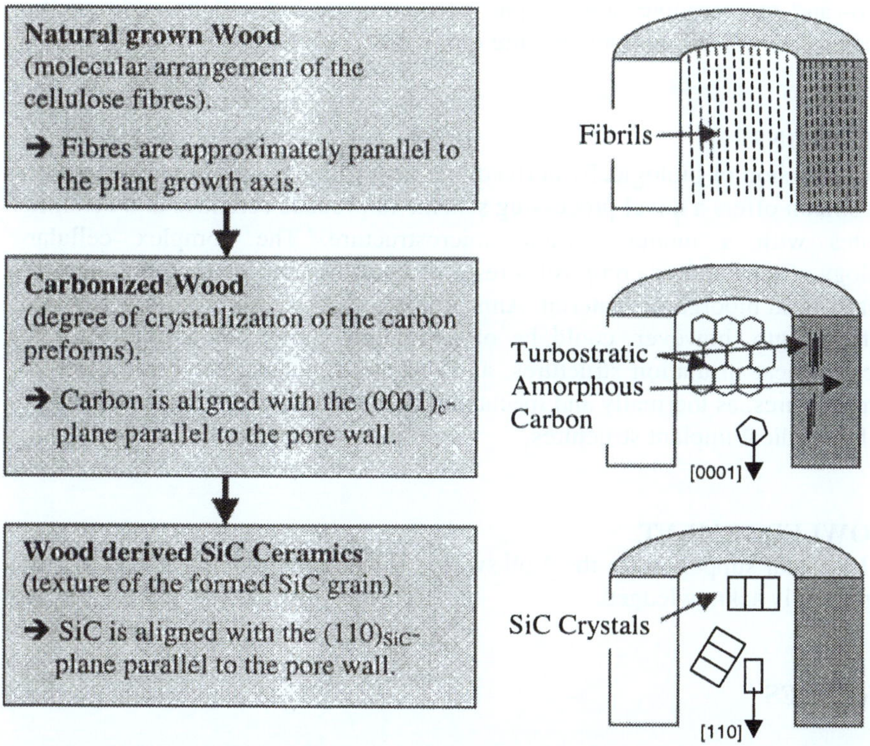

Fig. 7: Schematic sketch orientation relations during conversion of natural wood into SiC ceramics.

Results of the crystal orientation analysis by SEM/EBSD suggest that the SiC nucleation may be influenced by the orientation of pyrolyzed carbon structure in the pore surface (see Fig. 7). Wide angle X-ray spectroscopy and high-resolution SEM showed similar sheet like orientation of the basic structural units of polyaromatic carbon layers with the $[0001]_C$ direction perpendicular to the fibre elongation in carbon fibres derived from polyacrylnitril (PAN) and mesophase pitch-based carbon fibres [27,28]. It is suggested that the molecular orientation of the carbon induces a crystallographic texture of the formed ß-SiC.

A probable orientation relation was found to be $[110]_{SiC}$ // $[0001]_C$. The mechanical properties of such a cellular ceramic material will mainly depend on the meso- and macroscopic (anisotropic) pore structure but will be additionally influenced by the crystallographic texture of the matrix material.

CONCLUSIONS

Conversion of biologically derived preforms into SiC ceramic by liquid or gaseous silicon offers a novel processing scheme to produce ceramics and ceramic composites with a unique cellular microstructure. The complex cellular morphology of the ceramic composites result from different pore morphologies of the initially used bioorganic material. Anisotropic cellular ceramics of low density but high strength, however, could be of particular interest for applications in acoustic and heat insulation structures, as substrate, filter and catalyst carrier at high temperatures, as thermally and mechanically loaded light weight structures as well as for medical implant structures.

ACKNOWLEDGEMENT

Financial support from the Volkswagen Foundation under contract # I/73 043 is gratefully acknowledged.

REFERENCES

[1] A.H.Heuer, D.J.Fink, V.J.Laraia, J.L.Arias, P.D.Calvert, K.Kendali, G.L.Messing, J.Blackwell, P.C.Rieke, D.H.Thompson, A.P.Wheeler, A.Veis, A.I.Caplan, Innovative Material Processing Strategies: A Biomimetic Approach, Science **255** (1992) 1098.

[2] S.H.Li, Q.Y.Zeng, Y.L.Xiao, S.Y.Fu and B.L.Zhou, Biomimicry of bamboo bast fiber with engineering composite materials, Mat. Sci. Eng. **C3** (1995) 125.

[3] M.F. Ashby, On the Engineering Properties of Materials, Acta Metall. **37** (1989) 1273.

[4] M.F. Ashby, Materials and Shape, Acta Metall. **39** (1991) 1025.

[5] L.J. Gibson, Wood: A natural Fibre Reinforced Composite, Metals and Materials **8** (1992) 333.

[6] P.W. Lucas, B.W. Darvell, P.K. Lee, T.D.B. Yuen, M.F. Choong, The Toughness of Plant Cell Walls, Phil. Trans. Roy. Soc. Lond. **B 348** (1995) 363.

[7] L.J. Gibson, M.F. Ashby, Cellular Solids, Structure and Properties, Pergammon Press, New York (1988)

[8] R. Brezny, D.J. Green, Mechanical Behavior of cellular Ceramics, Chapter 9 in Mat. Sci. Techn. **11** VCH Verlag Weinheim/Germ. (1994) 463.

[9] P. Greil, T. Lifka, A. Kaindl, Biomorphic Silicon Carbide Ceramics from Wood: II. Mechanical Properties, J. Europ. Ceram. Soc. **18** (1998) 1974.

[10] I.A. Aksay, E. Baer, M. Sarikaya, D.A. Tirell (editors), Hierarchically Structured Materials, Mat. Res. Soc. Symp. Proc. Vol. **255** (1992) Mat. Res. Soc. Pittsburg/PE.

[11] M. Sarikaya, I.A. Aksay, An Introduction to Biomimetics: A Structural Viewpoint, in Microstructure of Materials, edited by K.M. Krishnan, San Francisco Press Inc., San Francisco/CA (1993).

[12] P. Calvert, Biomimetic Ceramic and Composites, Mat. Res. Soc. Bull. **17** (1992) 36

[13] T. Ota, M. Takahashi, T. Hibi, M. Ozawa, S. Suzuki, Y. Hikichi and H. Suzuki, Biomimetic Process for Producing SiC "Wood", J. Am. Ceram. Soc. **78** (1995) 3409.

[14] P. Greil, T. Lifka, A. Kaindl, Biomorphic Silicon Carbide Ceramics from Wood: I. Processing and Microstructure, J. Europ. Ceram. Soc. **18** (1998) 1961.

[15] M. Patel, B.K. Padhi, Production of Alumina Fibre through Jute Fibre Substrate, J.Mat.Sci. **25** (1990) 1335.

[16] M. Patel, B.K. Padhi, Titania Fibres through Jute Substrates, J. Mat. Sci. Lett. **12** (1993) 1234.

[17] R.V. Krishnaro, Y.R. Mahajan, Preparation of Silicon Carbide Fibres from Cotton Fibre and Silicon Nitride, J. Mat. Sci. Lett. **15** (1996) 232.

[18] R.V.Krishnarao, Y.R.Mahajan and T.J.Kumar, Conversion of Raw Rice Husk to SiC by Pyrolysis in Nitrogen Atmosphere, J. Europ. Cer. Soc. **18** (1998) 147.

[19] A.Selvan, N.G.Nair and P.Singh, Synthesis and characterization of SiC whisker from coconut shells, J. Mat. Sci. Let. **17** (1998) 57.

[20] W.B. Hillig, Melt Infiltration Approach to Ceramic Matrix Composites, J.Am.Ceram. Soc. **71** (1988) C 96.

[21] Y.M. Chiang, R.P. MEssner, C.D. Terwilliger, D.R. Behrendt, Reaction Formed Silicon Carbide, Mat.Sci.Eng. **A 144** (1991) 63.

[22] R. Pampuch, E. Walasek, J. Bialoskorski, Reaction Mechanism in Carbon-Liquid Silicon Systems at Elevated Temperatures, Ceram.Int. **12** (1986) 99.

[23] E. Fitzer, R. Gadow, Fibre-Reinforced Silicon-Carbide, Am. Ceram. Soc. Bull. **65** (1986) 326.

[24] T.J. Whalen, A.T. Anderson, Wetting of SiC, Si_3N_4, and Carbon by Si and Binary Si Alloys, J.Am.Ceram.Soc. **58** (1975) 396.

[25] S.C. Hardy, The Surface Tension of liquid Silicon, J. Crystal Growth **69** (1984) 456.

[26] L. Battezzati, A.L. Greer, The viscosity of liquid metals and alloys, Acta metall. **37** (1989) 1791.

[27] D.L. Vezie, W.W. Adams, High Resolution Scanning Electron Microscopy of PAN-based and Pitch-based Carbon Fibre, J. Mat. Sci. Let. **9** (1990) 883.

[28] S. Kumar, D.P. Anderson, A.S. Crasto, Carbon Fibre compressive Strength and its Dependence on Structure and Morphology, J. Mat. Sci. **28** (1993) 423.

SURFACE PROPERTIES OF LAYERED DOUBLE HYDROXIDE NANOCOMPOSITES

O. C. Wilson, Jr., T. Olorunyolemi, A. Jaworski, L. Borum, and D. Young
University of Maryland
Department of Materials and Nuclear Engineering
Building 090, Room 2130

E. Dickens
Eleanor Roosevelt High School
Greenbelt, MD 20770

C. Oriakhi
Hewlett Packard, OR

ABSTRACT

Mg and Al containing layered double hydroxides were synthesized with carbonate (LDHCO3), poly(styrenesulfonate) (LDHPSS) and poly(vinylsulfonate) (LDHPVS) inter-gallery species and characterized via X-ray diffraction (XRD), thermogravimetric analysis (TGA), Fourier transform infrared spectroscopy (FTIR), transmission electron microscopy (TEM), He pycnometry, and electrophoretic light scattering (ELS). Polymer incorporation was observed to increase the interlayer spacing and decrease the sample density as revealed by XRD and He pycnometry. While LDHCO3 exhibited an isoelectric point at pH 11, the LDH nanocomposites displayed a negative electrophoretic mobility over the measured pH range, indicating that the surface properties of the LDH nanocomposites were dominated by negatively charged sulfonate groups from adsorbed polymer molecules. This idea was further supported by the experimental observation that LDHCO3 suspensions that were equilibrated in the presence of poly(sodium styrene-4-sulfonate) displayed negative electrophoretic mobility values over the measured pH range of 6-11.

INTRODUCTION

Layered double hydroxides belong to a class of clay analogue materials that have received much attention in recent years. This interest stems from their wide range of current applications (catalysts, ceramic precursors, ion exchangers, pharmaceutical products, etc.) and their even wider range of potential applications. A big reason for the wider range of potential applications is due to the recent development of synthetic techniques to prepare LDH/polymer nanocomposies (1-3). Nanocomposites are particularly of interest because the electrical, mechanical, optical, and other physicochemical properties of the materials are often favorably modified due to nanometer level interphasic interactions and quantum effects (4, 5).

Layered double hydroxides (LDH) are composed of brucite-like (or gibbsite-like) M^{2+}, M^{3+} metal hydroxide layers which have a positive sheet charge that can be compensated by intercalation of simple or polymeric anions. As shown in Figure 1 for a Mg/Al LDH, the substitution of Al^{3+} in the lattice results in a positive charge on the sheet. The incorporation of different anions in the gallery region causes changes in both the gallery height and the interlayer spacing. While carbonate anions are preferentially adsorbed in the interlayer or gallery region due to their small size and charge, relatively large polymer molecules can be intercalated in the gallery region if carbonate is excluded. Because of these unique features, LDH possess interesting layer and interlayer chemistry that can be tailored to accommodate a wide range of sheet compositions and interlayer species for various developmental uses.

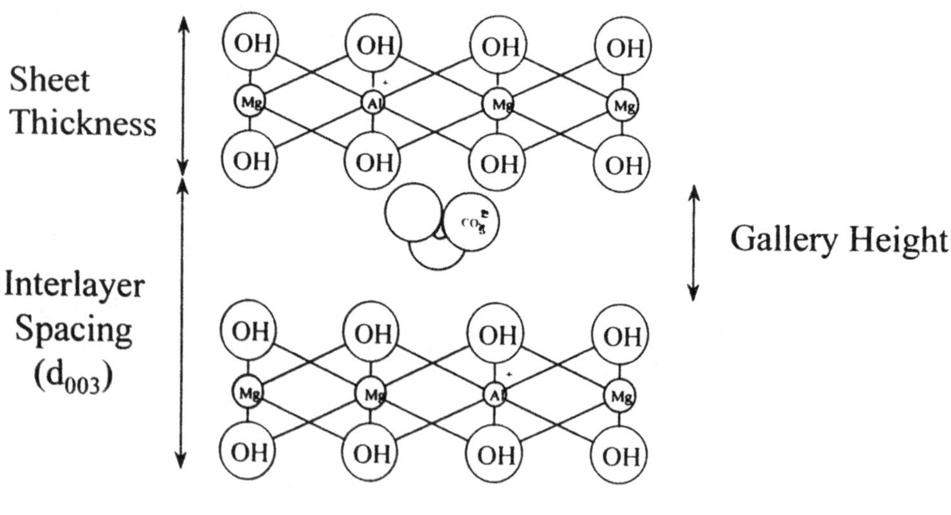

Figure 1. Schematic diagram of LDH.

The development of LDH nanocomposites with biomedical applications is a very interesting topic that has been recently reported. Whilton et al. (3) synthesized bioinorganic clays by intercalating poly(amino acids) within the gallery region of LDH. Others have reported attempts to intercalate drugs in LDH for the development of controlled release drug delivery systems (6). Another very interesting possibility for LDH nanocomposites is in the development of novel biocomposites. By choosing appropriate polymer compositions for the interlayer phase and the matrix, very versatile composites with very small levels of mixing (nanocomposite particles within a polymer composite matrix) can be synthesized and used for a wide variety of potential biomaterial applications. The following report focuses on characterization data for LDH nanocomposites containing poly(vinylsulfonate) and poly(sodium styrene-4-sulfonate) with an emphasis on the influence of polymer macromolecules on the electrophoretic mobility of the composites.

EXPERIMENTAL PROCEDURES

Chemical Reagents

All reagents used in this work were of analytical grade and used without further purification. Poly(sodium styrene-4-sulfonate) (PSS, Mw = 70,000) and poly(sodium vinylsulfonate) (PVS, 25 wt% in water, Mw = 40,000 to 60,000) were used as received from Aldrich Chemical Company. Doubly distilled and/or de-ionized water was used for preparation of all solutions.

LDH Synthesis

Syntheses of carbonate-containing LDH (LDH2CO3 and LDH3CO3): The LDH containing interlayer carbonate with Mg/Al ratios of 2:1 (LDH2CO3) and 3:1 (LDH3CO3) were prepared following a standard aqueous co-precipitation and thermal crystallization method (7). The following procedure was typically used to synthesize LDH3CO3. A stoichiometric amount of $Mg(NO_3)_2.6H_2O$ (3.93 g, 0.015 mol) and $Al(NO_3)_3.9H_2O$ (1.85 g, 0.005 mol) in 50-100 ml of water was slowly added to 100 ml of a solution containing NaOH (3.00 g, 0.075 mol) and Na_2CO_3 (2.34 g, 0.022 mol). The resulting gelatinous precipitate was aged at 65 °C for 24 h, filtered and washed with large quantities of water until the pH of the supernatant solution was neutral. The powder was dried in air at room temperature for 24 hr.

Synthesis of PSS and PVS-containing LDHs (LDHPSS and LDHPVS): Polymer containing LDH nanocomposites were prepared following the template method (2). De-aerated solutions of mixed metal nitrate and NaOH were simultaneously added to a basic solution of the polymer. The reaction was performed under a nitrogen atmosphere to prevent preferential intercalation of carbonate in the presence of CO_2. In a typical synthesis, 2.5 g of PSS or PVS was dissolved in 100 g of N_2-purged water in a three-necked flask and solutions of $Mg(NO_3)_2.6H_2O$ (4.80 g, 0.018 mol), $Al(NO_3)_3.9H_2O$ (2.34 g, 0.0062 mol) and NaOH (3.00 g, 0.075 mol) were slowly added simultaneously while stirring. The resulting gel was aged at 65 °C for 24 hr and was filtered, washed several times with hot water to remove excess polymer, and dried under vacuum for 24 hr.

Characterization

X-ray diffraction (XRD) patterns were recorded for the LDH nanocomposite samples using a Siemens D5000 powder diffractometer with Ni-filtered Cu Kα radiation (λ = 0.154 nm). Data were collected over the angular range from 2-60° 2θ in increments of 0.02 °/sec at room temperature. Thermal gravimetric analysis (TGA) was performed for the carbonate, PSS, and PVS forms of the LDH using a Schimadzu TGA-50 Thermogravimetric Analyzer (Kyoto, Japan). Samples (20-24 mg) were ground in a mortar and pestle and placed in an alumina sample pan. All samples were heated in air at a rate of 10 °C/min to a temperature of 1000-1050 °C. Fourier transform infrared (FTIR) analysis was performed using a Nicolet 500 Series optical bench and a diffuse reflectance measuring cell. Samples were prepared by mixing LDH powders with optical spectra grade KBr in the proper ratio to obtain 10 wt% of LDH sample. Sample spectra were collected over the range of 4000-400 cm^{-1} and were averaged over a minimum of 36 scans. Density measurements were performed using a Micromeritics model 1305 Multi-volume He Pycnometer (Norcross, GA). The density data was found to be very sensitive to the sample drying method. In order to avoid errors from the loss of structural water that occurs on drying at elevated temperatures (up to 120 °C), LDH nanocomposites were vacuum dried overnight at room temperature prior to density determination. Transmission electron microscopy (TEM) analysis was performed using a Hitachi model H-600AB electron microscope (San Jose, CA). TEM samples were prepared by dipping amorphous carbon coated copper TEM grids into dilute aqueous or ethanol suspensions of the LDH powders. The TEM grids were allowed to dry in air before analysis. Samples were imaged at an accelerating voltage of 100 KV.

The electrophoretic mobility (μ) of LDH composites was measured using a Malvern Zetasizer 3000 (Malvern, England) with a flow through sample cell and software version 1.34. Samples were prepared by dispersing 0.005 vol% of each LDH nanocomposite powder in 0.005 M $NaNO_3$ in polypropylene sample cups. The pH of individual samples was adjusted with NaOH and HNO_3 to cover the range from 4-12. In order to provide a comparison for the LDH polymer intercalated nanocomposite samples, a number of LDH2CO3 samples were prepared by aging 0.005 vol% LDH2CO3 in 0.005 M $NaNO_3$ at different pHs in the presence of 1 g/L PSS. Electrophoretic mobility measurements were performed at 25 °C after the samples were allowed to equilibrate overnight. The μ of the LDH powders was measured at the stationary plane using the technique of electrophoretic light scattering. Each data point depicted in the μ vs. pH plot (Figure 4) represents the mean of 3-5 separate analysis runs. The error bars for each sample represent the maximum standard deviation that was obtained for any particular data point in each series.

RESULTS AND DISCUSSION

A summary of the XRD, density, and TGA data for the LDH nanocomposite samples is shown in Table 1. The LDH samples with interlayer carbonate displayed a peak that was attributed to reflections from the {003} crystallographic planes (Figure 1). This interlayer spacing (termed d_{003} for one-third of the unit cell dimension in the c direction) is determined by the sheet thickness (~ 0.48 nm) and the gallery region that contains intercalated carbonate anions (~ 0.28 nm). Intercalation of larger polymer molecules such as PSS and PVS between the LDH sheets resulted in an increase in the interlayer spacing. Compared to the d_{003} reflections for LDH2CO3 and LDH3CO3 (0.77 nm), the corresponding interlayer spacing for LDHPVS and LDHPSS shifted to 1.27 and 2.1 nm, respectively.

Table 1. Layer spacing, density and TGA data for LDH nanocomposites

Sample	d003 (nm)	ρ (g/cm^3)	TGA (wt loss%)
LDH3CO3	0.77	2.05	42.1
LDH2CO3	0.77	------	43.5
LDHPVS	1.27	1.83	55.1
LDHPSS	2.10	1.41	59.9

Polymer intercalation also resulted in a change in density that was inversely related to the polymer molecule size. The density values for LDHPVS and LDHPSS were measured as 1.83 g/cm^3 and 1.41 g/cm^3. The decrease in density can be attributed to the increased interlayer spacing that is filled with a low-density polymer phase. Vichi and Alves (8) used density measurements to show how the incorporation of phenylphosphonic acid and 2 carboxyethylphosphonic acid decreased the density of Cd/Al LDH from 2.66 g/cm^3 (for the nitrate containing

Cd/Al LDH) to 1.24 g/cm^3 for the LDH with intercalated 2 carboxyethylphosphonic acid.

The TGA weight loss values for the LDH samples revealed larger weight loss values for the polymer containing samples. The TGA weight loss for sample LDH2CO3 was typical for LDH materials with interlayer carbonate. However, sample LDH3CO3 displayed different features that indicated a potential impurity phase. The total weight loss for this sample (42.1 wt%) was slightly less than the weight loss for carbonate LDHs with a Mg/Al ratio of 3:1 (43.1 wt%) as reported by Puttaswamy and Kamath (9). In addition, an uncharacteristic weight loss of approximately 8 wt% occurred above 800 °C.

FTIR spectra for samples LDH2CO3, LDH3CO3, LDHPVS, and LDHPSS are shown in Figure 2. All four samples displayed similar features due to water and hydroxyl vibrational modes in the region between 4000-1600 cm^{-1}. OH stretching caused a very strong and broad absorption band at approximately 3590 cm^{-1}. Del Arco et al. (10) attributed the broadness of the hydroxyl stretch region to the presence

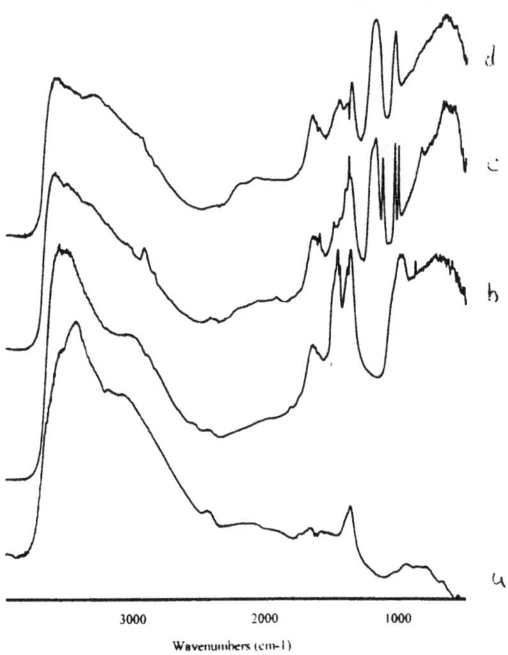

Figure 2 FTIR spectra for a.) LDH2CO3, b.) LDH3CO3, c.) LDHPSS, and d.) LDHPVS

of hydrogen bonded hydroxyl groups. The absorption band at 1650-1655 cm^{-1} was attributed to a δ(HOH) bending mode for water. Spectral features below

1600 cm^{-1} were due to the interlayer species carbonate, PVS, and PSS. The polymer containing LDH samples displayed peaks that are consistent with the incorporation of sulfonated polymers. Both LDHVS and LDHPSS displayed sharp peaks at 1196 and 1040 cm^{-1} which are characteristic of S-O vibrations (in RSO_3 species).

Comparison of the spectral features for the carbonate containing LDH samples revealed that sample LDH3CO3 did contain a carbonate impurity phase based on the following analysis. The free carbonate anion possesses D_{3h} symmetry and gives rise to the ν_1 (C-O symmetrical stretch at 1065 cm^{-1}), ν_2 (the carbonate out of plane deformation at 880 cm^{-1}), ν_3 (C-O asymmetrical stretch at 1400 cm^{-1}), and the ν_4 (the carbonate in plane (rocking) deformation at 685 cm^{-1}) vibrational modes (11). Shifts in these modes should reflect positional constraints or specific coordination of carbonate anions. The FTIR data for both LDH2CO3 and LDH3CO3 displayed a srong peak at 1369 with a weak split at 1390 cm^{-1}. The bands at 1369 and 1390 cm^{-1} were attributed to the carbonate stretching mode (ν_3) and have been observed for other carbonate containing LDH samples (2, 10). However, LDH3CO3 displayed two additional peaks that indicated the presence of carbonate in a different coordination state. The additional bands at 1449 and 1463 cm^{-1} (with slight shoulders at 1483 and 1503 cm^{-1}) may also be attributed to ν_3 carbonate-stretching modes based on the similarity with ν_3 modes obtained for $CuCO_3$ at 1460 and 1420 cm^{-1} (12). A reference sample of $MgCO_3$ displayed 2 strong bands at 1424 and 1483 cm^{-1} with a shoulder at 1509 cm^{-1}. These results indicated that two types of carbonate (interlayer carbonate and carbonate associated with metal cations in LDH sheets) existed in sample LDH3CO3. Compared to the free carbonate anion, interlayer containment shifted the ν_3 carbonate mode to lower frequencies while coordination with metal cations shifted the ν_3 carbonate mode to higher frequencies.

The electrophoretic mobility (μ) vs. pH data for the LDH samples is displayed in Figure 3. Both samples LDH2CO3 and LDH3CO3 exhibited both positive and negative μ regions that were separated by an isoelectric point (iep) that occurred near pH 11. The μ vs. pH plot for both carbonate containing samples were closely related with differences in specific regions attributable to differences in the Mg/Al ratio and the carbonate impurity phase. The insertion of polymers into LDH resulted in notable differences in the μ vs. pH behavior of LDH nanocomposites. Samples LDHPVS and LDHPSS exhibited a negative μ for the pH range 4-12 with no iep. The μ data for LDHPSS varied between -2.9 x 10^{-8} m^2/Vs to -4.0 x 10^{-8} m^2/Vs and was slightly more negative than the data for LDHPVS. The μ for LDHPVS decreased from a value of -1.5 x 10^{-8} m^2/Vs at pH 4 to -3.35 x 10^{-8} m^2/Vs at pH 11.2. Extrapolation of the μ data for LDHPVS would yield an iep at pH 2-3. However, all LDH samples were observed to dissolve when the solution pH was below 4.

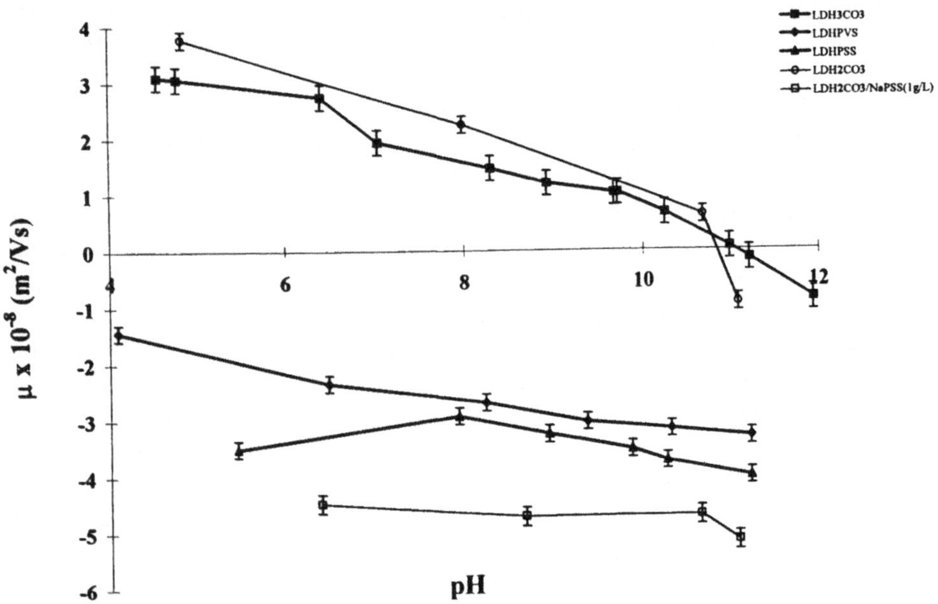

Figure 3. Electrophoretic mobility vs. pH data for LDH samples (0.005 vol% solids loading, 0.005 M $NaNO_3$.

The μ vs. pH data for the polymer containing nanocomposites is very similar to data reported for sulfonated polystyrene latex. Bastos et al. (13) used sodium styrene sulfonate monomer to synthesize polystyrene latex particles with sulfonate surface sites. After extensive washing, the μ of the polystyrene latex was found to be approximately -5 to -6 x 10^{-8} m^2/Vs over the pH range 2-12. The similarity between the μ for the sulfonated polystyrene latex and the LDH nanocomposites indicates that the nanocomposites have sulfonate sites in the near surface region.The μ vs. pH data for the polymer containing nanocomposites is very similar to data reported for sulfonated polystyrene latex. Bastos et al. (13) used sodium styrene sulfonate monomer to synthesize polystyrene latex particles with sulfonate surface sites. After extensive washing, the μ of the polystyrene latex was found to be approximately -5 to -6 x 10^{-8} m^2/Vs over the pH range 2-12. The similarity between the μ for the sulfonated polystyrene latex and the LDH nanocomposites indicates that the nanocomposites have sulfonate sites in the near surface region.

The influence of PSS adsorption on the μ of LDH2CO3 was further evaluated by aging 0.005 vol% suspensions of LDH2CO3 in 0.005 M $NaNO_3$ in the presence of 1 g/L PSS. The mobility values that were measured for these samples shifted to negative values that were even lower than the values for the polymer containing nanocomposite samples (Figure 3). This result shows that anionic polymers have a strong affinity for adsorbing onto the surface of LDH materials and indicates that surface adsorbed anionic polymer contributed to the negative mobility results that were obtained for the polymer containing nanocomposites. Another factor that substantiates this idea is the presence of excess polymer in solution during the formation and charge stabilization of the LDH nanocomposites. Calculations show that over three times as much polymer was present in solution than the amount required to counteract the LDH sheet charge. The excess polymer would be available in solution to adsorb onto the surface of the LDH nanocomposites and contribute to the μ behavior of the LDH nanocomposites. This result has strong implications for evaluating the influence of polymer molecules on the nucleation and growth processes that occur during the formation and charge stabilization of LDH nanocomposites (14).

CONCLUSIONS

The intercalation of polymer molecules in LDH nanocomposites was revealed by an increase in the interlayer spacing and a decrease in the density. Polymer adsorption/intercalation also influenced the electrokinetic behavior of LDH nanocomposites as revealed by a shift of the μ to more negative values. This behavior can be attributed to both intercalated polymer molecules and surface adsorbed polymer molecules with sulfonate surface groups.

REFERENCES

1) Messersmith, P. B., and Stupp, S. I., "Synthesis of Nanocomposites: Organoceramics," J. Mater. Res., 7, 2599-2611 (1992).

2) Oriakhi, C. O., Farr, I. V., and Lerner, M., "Incorporation of Poly(acrylic acid), Poly(vinylsulfonate), and Poly(styrenesulfonate) within Layered Double Hydroxides," J. Mater. Chem., 6(1) 103-107 (1996).

3) Whilton, N. T., Vickers, P. J., and Mann, S., Bioinorganic Clays: Synthesis and Characterization of Amino- and Polyamino Acid Intercalated Layered Double Hydroxides," J. Mater. Chem., 7(8) 1623-1629 (1997).

4) Komarneni, S., "Nanocomposites," J. Mater. Chem., 2, 1219-1230 (1992).

5) Ozin, G. A., "Nanochemistry: Synthesis in Diminishing Dimensions," Adv. Mater., 4, 612-649 (1992).

6) Carlino, S., "Chemistry Between the Sheets," Chem. Brit., 33, 59-62 (1997).

7) Riechle, W. T., "Catalytic Reactions by Thermally Activated Synthetic Anionic Clay Minerals," J. Catal., 94, 547-557 (1985).

8) Vichi, F. M. and Alves, O. L., "Preparation of Cd/Al Layered Double Hydroxides and their Intercalation Reactions with Phosphonic Acids," J. Mater. Chem., 7(8) 1631-1634 (1997).

9) Puttaswamy, N. S. and Kamath, P. V., "Reversible Thermal Behavior of Layered Double Hydroxides: A Thermogravimetric Study," J. Mater. Chem. 7(9) 1941-1945 (1997).

10) del Arco, M., Martin, C., Martin, I., Rives, V., and Trulillano, R., "A FTIR Spectroscopic Study of Surface Acidity and Basicity of Mixed Mg, Al-Oxides Obtained by Thermal Decomposition of Hydrotalcite," Spectrochimica Acta, 49A(11) 1575-1582 (1993).

11) Palmer, D. A. and Van Eldik, R., "The Chemistry of Metal Carbonato and Carbon Dioxide Complexes," Chem. Rev., 83, 651-731 (1983).

12) Seidel, V. H., Viswanathan, K., Johannes, W., and Ehrhardt, H.. "Synthesis, Structure, and Properties of Cupric Carbonate," Z. Anorg. Allg. Chem., 410, 138-148 (1974).

13) Bastos, D., de las Nieves, F.J., "Effect of Electrolyte Type on the Electrokinetic Behavior of Sulfonated Polystyrene Model Colloids," Colloid Polym. Sci., 271, 860-867 (1993).

14) Wilson, Jr., O. C., Olorunyolemi, T., Jaworski, A., Borum, L., Young, D., Siriwat, A., Dickens, E., Oriakhi, C., and Lerner, M., "Surface and Interfacial Properties of Polymer-Intercalated Layered Double Hydroxide Nanocomposites," (accepted for publication in Applied Clay Science).

NEAR-NET-SHAPE FORMING TECHNIQUE FOR BIOCERAMIC COMPONENTS

A. Salomoni, I. Stamenkovic, L. Esposito and A. Tucci
Italian Ceramic Center
Via Martelli, 26
40138 Bologna, ITALY

ABSTRACT

Several mixtures of alumina and partially stabilised zirconia high purity powders were characterised and used to study processing routes for the fabrication of high performance implant components. The powders were used to make highly loaded, well dispersed, stable suspensions of low viscosity. High pressure casting, from 2 to 10 MPa, was employed to prepare suitable specimens from the slips deemed most appropriate. The casting kinetics and the roles of specific processing parameters are evaluated. The as cast bodies are characterised by homogeneous microstructure and the fired ones by submicronic grains. The mixture with the best performances, in comparison to alumina used as a reference material, was chosen on the basis of the bending strength, fracture toughness and results of pin-on-disc wear tests. With this mixture, near-net-shape prototypes were produced using the developed processing technique and then characterised. Aspects regarding the practical use of pressure slip casting, to fabricate high quality products and significantly reduce the machining operations, are discussed.

INTRODUCTION

Ceramic materials are widely used for the repair and reconstruction of damaged parts of the skeletal system[1]. In particular, during the last two decades, successful surgical total hip joint replacements are mainly due to the widespread use of bioceramics. Alumina is the material most often employed in total hip prosthesis because of its favourable combination of chemical inertness, good biocompatibility, high strength and high wear resistance[2]. It has been used in orthopaedic surgery for more than 20 years[3]. The considerable effort, directed towards improving its mechanical characteristics have led to a new generation of aluminas with exceptionally low coefficients of friction and minimal wear rates[2,4]. Nevertheless, the too high Young's modulus of alumina and its low fracture toughness still represent a failure risk that must be reduced[5].

In the last few years, medical-grade zirconia ceramics have been developed for use in total hip joint prostheses[6]. These materials are inert in the physiological environment and are characterised by a higher fracture toughness and tensile strength and lower Young's modulus thus showing net advantages over alumina, according to some authors[7]. On the other hand, the lower hardness and wear resistance, in comparison with alumina, still represent important limitations that negatively affect the service life of zirconia implants[2].

To overcome these intrinsic drawbacks and taking into account the basic concepts of ceramic composites[8], the development of a new composite material for biomedical components may become a viable solution. In particular, alumina-zirconia composites may represent such a material, since their good mechanical characteristics are indicative of their high potential. However, forming and densification of multiphase ceramics present serious problems due to the low particle packing levels of the green bodies and inadequate adhesion among the single components. Close control of the microstructure is fundamental to improve the mechanical properties and reliability of a ceramic component. The necessity to obtain highly densified bodies with submicronic grains and a narrow grain size distribution, obliges the use of both very fine and pure starting powders, as well as the most appropriate forming technique and firing cycle. Submicronic powders are usually strongly agglomerated and the manufacturing technologies require the elimination of agglomerates, the presence of which unavoidably creates macropores during sintering.

Colloidal processes are able to overcome these problems, eliminating the majority of microstructural dishomogeneities, that may be introduced by powders. Indeed, pressure slip casting (PSC) of well dispersed aqueous suspensions of submicronic and agglomerated powders has given high level results[9]. This forming technique makes it possible to obtain near-net shape bodies with a homogeneous microstructure, from which reliable components can be produced that are also economically attractive.

The present investigation was focused on the aspects and implications related to the forming of near-net-shape bioceramic components using several mixtures of alumina-zirconia powders. A significant part of the investigation regards the physical-mechanical characterisation of the as shaped and sintered materials and the wear responses of the components.

EXPERIMENTAL

The following powders were studied: two single oxides, an alumina A (SM8, Baikowski, France), and a 3 mol% yttria stabilised zirconia Z (TZ 3YS, TOSOH, Japan) and four oxide mixtures (all supplied by TOSOH, Japan) with different ratioes of alumina and 3 mol% yttria stabilised zirconia, denoted 8Z2A (TZ 3Y20A), 6Z4A (TZ 3Y40A), 4Z6A (TZ 3Y60A) and 2Z8A (TZ 3Y80A). The characteristic properties of these materials are reported in Table I.

These powders are characterised by high purity and sinterability. Their contents of SiO_2+CaO+alkalies range between 0.005 and 0.019 wt%, well below the requirement of the ISO 6474-92 standard ($\leq$ 0.1 wt%).

Different slips were prepared by mixing water, dispersant (a polycarbonic acid free of alkalies) and powder in a centrifugal mill (zirconia jar and balls) and then characterised. Particular attention was paid to their rheological behaviour through viscosity and yield stress measurements carried out using a rotational rheometer (mod. RS 50, HAAKE, Germany).

Table I. Characteristics of the starting powders

Powder	Composition, wt%		Surface area, m^2/g	Particle size, µm		Agglomerate size, µm
	ZrO_2	Al_2O_3		ZrO_2	Al_2O_3	
Z	100	0	7	0.2	---	8 - 85
8Z2A	80	20	16	< 0.1	< 0.3	10 - 100
6Z4A	60	40	15	< 0.3	< 0.3	8 - 75
4Z6A	40	60	12	< 0.3	< 0.3	10 - 80
2Z8A	20	80	10	< 0.1	< 0.3	10 - 80
A	0	100	10	---	0.2	5 - 170

The optimised slips were then densified by pressure casting using a laboratory device especially developed for this purpose[10], Figure 1.

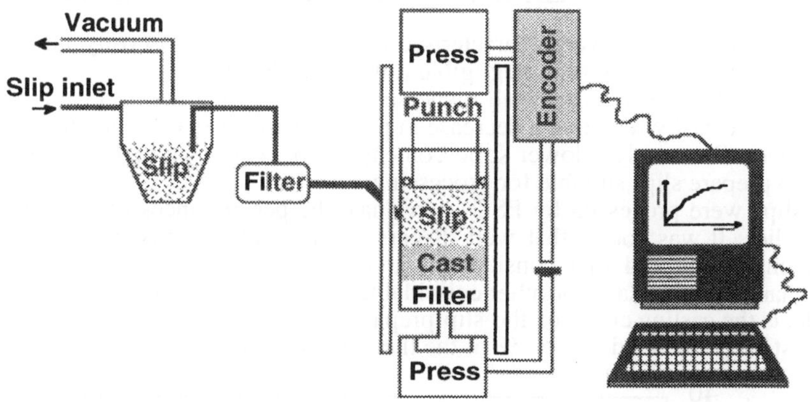

Fig. 1. Scheme of the laboratory pressure slip casting device

This device permitted continuous recording of the green body thickness, casting time and pressures making it possible to obtain the casting curves vs. time, in function of the pressure.

The influence of the pressure (over the range 1.7 to 10.0 MPa) and time (up to 60 min) was studied during PSC of the green bodies having different geometries (discs, spheres, tubes) and thicknesses (15 to 50 mm).

The pressure cast samples were sintered in air, at temperatures ranging from 1500 °C to 1600 °C depending on their composition, to allow them to reach theoretical density. The morphological and mechanical characterisation of the fired samples has been described in more detail elsewhere[10-12].

The tribological behaviour of the materials studied was examined by a "pin-on-disc" apparatus at the following test parameters: dry condition, room temperature, 33 N normal load and 1.0 m/s sliding speed.

RESULTS AND DISCUSSION

The characteristics of the optimised slips are reported in Table II.

Table II. Characteristics of the optimised slips

Slip	Solid content	Dispersant content	pH	Viscosity (at D=500 s^{-1})	Particle size (d_{50})
	vol%	wt% of powder		mPa s	µm
Z	33.0	0.3	8.7	16.2	0.54
8Z2A	21.0	1.8	9.1	11.5	0.57
6Z4A	33.0	0.6	8.9	14.9	0.42
4Z6A	24.6	0.8	9.1	16.7	n. d.
2Z8A	33.0	0.4	9.1	9.2	0.51
A	43.0	0.5	9.4	16.4	0.48

All the slips prepared were characterised by low values of viscosity and yield stress, pseudoplastic behaviour, negligible time-dependency.

This means that the slips are well dispersed. By comparing the data of Tables I and II it can be easily seen that a decrease in powder particle size, i.e. an increase in surface area, allows only a lower solid content and/or requires a higher dispersant content to prepare slips suitable for processing.

The slips were processed by PSC to evaluate the performances of so obtained green bodies. It was found that well dispersed slips produce cast bodies with a high green density and that considerable thicknesses can be attained in a time shorter than that necessary for other colloidal techniques. Shown in Figure 2, as an example, is the casting curve of the slip prepared with 6Z4A powder. The density of the cast body obtained was 53 % of the theoretical density.

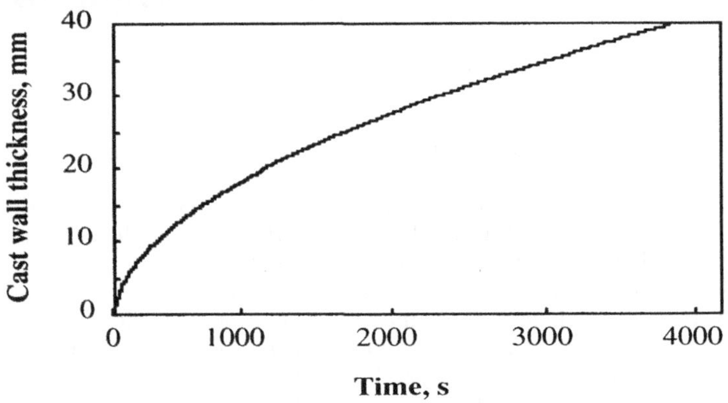

Fig. 2. Pressure casting curve of the 6Z4A slip at 5.6 MPa

On the basis of both casting parameters and characteristics of densified samples, the most advantageous forming parameters were chosen for further experimentation.

The cast bodies were sintered and microstructural and physical characterisation of the sintered bodies was carried out. The most relevant results are reported in Table III and in Figure 3 a, b and c.

Table III. Physical-microstructural characteristics of the sintered materials

Material	Density g/cm^3	Mean grain size µm	
		ZrO_2	Al_2O_3
Z	6.05	0.63	----
8Z2A	5.48	0.38	0.49
6Z4A	5.02	0.27	0.50
4Z6A	4.60	0.24	0.42
2Z8A	4.27	0.25	0.62
A	3.95	----	1.27

All the samples reached theoretical density and show a homogeneous microstructure, characterised by submicronic and equiaxed grains. Higher sintering temperatures generally lead to alumina grain growth. Abnormal growth of alumina, however was never observed. X-ray diffraction analysis of the sintered samples confirmed the presence of α-alumina and zirconia, always in its tetragonal phase.

The mechanical characteristics of the sintered materials are reported in Table IV.

Table IV. Mechanical characteristics of the sintered materials

Material	Bending strength*, MPa	Weibull's modulus	Young's modulus GPa	Hardness HV_{20}, GPa	K_{IC}° MPa $\sqrt{m}$
Z	766	11.7	205	13.3	5.9
8Z2A	811	13.3	246	14.3	6.4
6Z4A	912	7.3	285	15.1	6.9
4Z6A	834	11.4	316	16.4	4.6
2Z8A	717	7.7	348	17.8	4.6
A	436	9.7	356	18.3	5.7

*Four point bending test
°Vickers indentation method

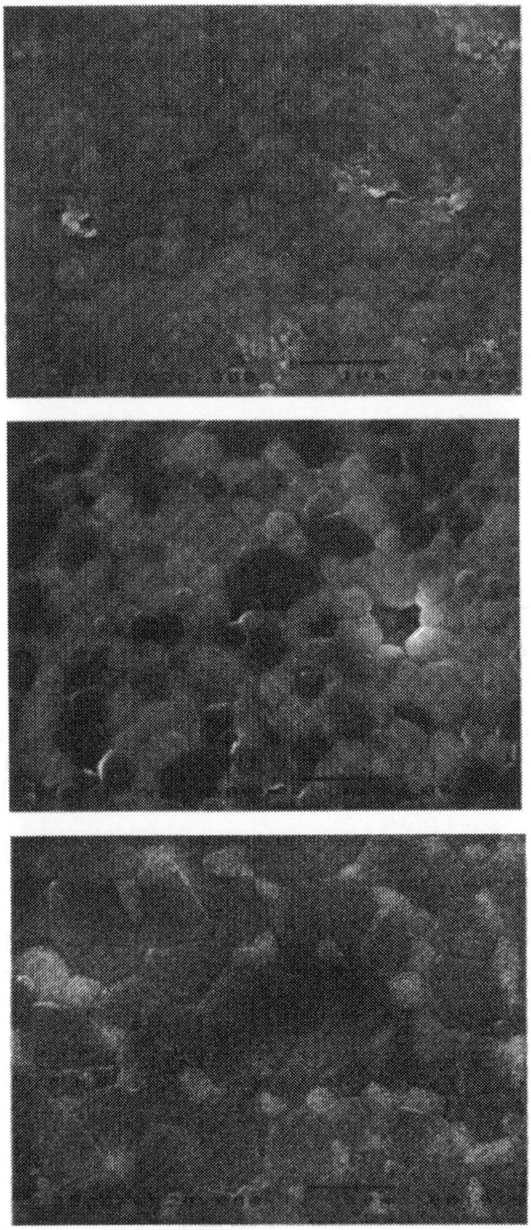

Fig. 3. SEM micrographs of the microstructures: a) Z, b) 6Z4A and c) 2Z8A

It is interesting to note that the bending strength of the samples containing zirconia is considerably higher than that of material A. The maximum value of 912 MPa is reached with the composite 6Z4A. As expected, both Young's modulus and hardness increase when the zirconia content decreases. Toughness however is not directly related to the zirconia content. In fact, the highest K_{IC} value is shown by the composite 6Z4A and the toughness of the Z material is only slightly higher than that of the A material. This behaviour can be explained through the particular microstructure of the studied zirconia which consisted of very small, round grains, that cause only a limited induced transformation zone, and consequently a rather low toughening effect[13]. Furthermore, as previously reported[14], the addition of alumina to a zirconia matrix induces the formation of a highly toughened alumina-zirconia grain boundary, that strongly contrasts crack propagation, favouring an increase in both toughness and strength of the composite. This effect appears to reach its maximum in the case of the 6Z4A material.

The results of the tribological tests carried out on the entire series of samples, tested against a reference material (a high purity alumina pin) are given in Figure 4.

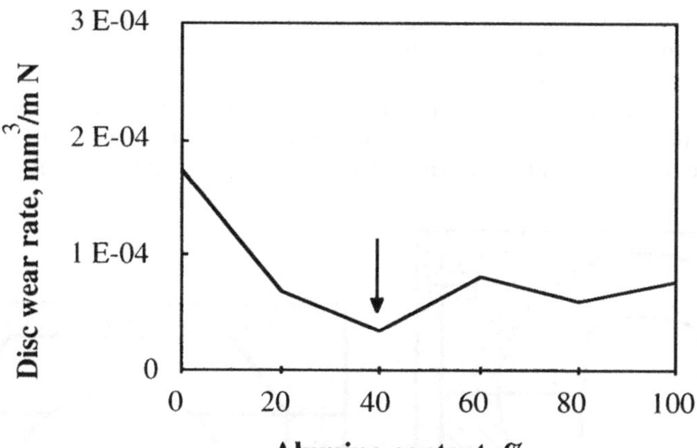

Fig. 4. Wear rate of the sintered materials as a function of their alumina content

With increasing alumina content of the specimens, the wear rate initially decreases, reaching its lowest value with the 6Z4A material, and then shows a slight increase.

SEM observations of the worn surfaces show that fracture constitutes the main wear mechanism involved. The lowest wear rate shown by the 6Z4A material is essentially due to its good mechanical properties in terms of strength and fracture toughness, which are the best of all the materials studied.

The relatively low value of Weibull's modulus of this material indicates that its preparation procedure could be further improved.

DEVELOPMENT OF ZIRCONIA-ALUMINA BIOCOMPONENTS

On the basis of the results obtained it was decided to make a series of hip joint components prototypes to evaluate the feasibility of the process studied for production on an industrial scale.

A flow sheet for the production of the hip joint prosthesis components was set up using the optimised slip prepared with the 6Z4A powder.

One of the first problems faced to produce near-net shape green bodies was to design and manufacture suitable moulds for PSC processing of the chosen slip. Several approaches in designing the moulds, and choosing materials for making them were evaluated. The objectives were to improve the shaping procedure, reduce scrap and allow shorter casting times. Near-net-shape moulds, made from stainless steel and porous resin, as shown in Figure 5, have been designed and realised. Several series of prototypes of femoral heads and acetabular cups were produced using the laboratory pressure casting device equipped with these moulds.

The machining operations, performed in two steps after prefiring and after sintering, were optimised by an Italian company.

It is worth noting that, by using these moulds and the process developed, it was possible to reduce the total production costs by about 40%, due to the substantial reduction in processing and machining operations on the green bodies and final components having already near-net- shape.

After sintering, the prototypes were thoroughly tested by the techniques typical for this field, to evaluate their biochemical and mechanical performances, and by a hip-joint simulator, to evaluate their wear response. The results of these tests confirmed those already obtained during characterisation of the materials.

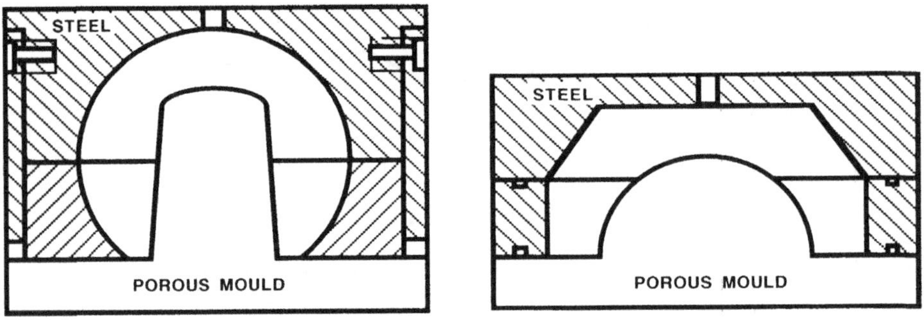

Fig. 5. Schemes of the near net shape moulds used for pressure casting of a hip prosthesis head and acetabular cup

CONCLUSIONS

New ceramic biomaterials were studied together with a new technology to produce components for hip joint prostheses.

A series of highly sinterable powders with a different ratio of TZP and alumina was characterised and used. A procedure for the preparation of suspensions was developed. A laboratory pressure slip casting device was designed and assembled to study the kinetics and optimise the suspension for colloidal shaping.

On the basis of the characteristic properties of green and sintered samples, such as microstructural homogeneity, bending strength, hardness, fracture toughness and wear resistance, the material 6Z4A (60 wt% Y-TZP + 40 wt% alumina) was selected for the production of biomedical implants.

Based on the laboratory results, a flow sheet for the production of hip joint prosthesis components was set up. Prosthesis heads and acetabular cups were prepared and characterised. Their mechanical and microstructural parameters reached the expected, very high levels.

REFERENCES

[1]L.L. Hench "Bioceramics", *Journal of the American Ceramic Society* , 81[7] 1705-1728 (1998).

[2]S.F. Hulbert "The Use of Alumina and Zirconia in Surgical Implants", pp. 41-62 in *An Introduction of Bioceramics*, Edited by L.L. Hench and J. Wilson. World Scientific Publishing, Singapore 1993.

[3]S.F. Hulbert, J.C. Bokros, L.L. Hench, J. Wilson and G. Heimke "Ceramic in Clinical Applications - Past, Present and Future", pp. 3-27 in *Ceramic in Clinical Application*, Edited by P. Vincenzini. Elsevier, Amsterdam 1987.

[4]H.G. Richter and G. Willmann "Reliability of Ceramic Components for Total Hip Endoprostheses", *British Ceramic Transactions* , 98[1] 29-34 (1999).

[5]P.E. Thorne "Influence of Zirconia on Hip Prosthesis Coupling Systems"; p. 122 in *Hip Prosthetic Coupling: Certainties, Illusions and Hopes*, Proceeding International Symposium. Vignola-Bologna, 1992.

[6]G. Burger and G.Willman "Advantages and Risks of Zirconia Ceramics in Biomedical Application", pp. 299-304 in *BIOCERAMICS*, Edited by P. Ducheyne and D. Christiansen. Butterworth-Heinmann Publication 1993.

[7]R.M. Streicher, M. Semlitsch and R. Schon "Articulation of Ceramic Surfaces against Polyethylene", pp. 118-123 in *Bioceramics and Human Body*, Edited by A. Ravaglioli and A. Krajewski. Elsevier Applied Science, London 1991.

[8]A.G. Evans "Perspective on the Development of High-Toughness Ceramics", *Journal of the American Ceramic Society* , 73[2] 187-206 (1990).

[9]S.M. Castanho, R. Moreno, A. Salomoni and I. Stamenkovic, "Slip Casting and Pressure Slip Casting of Si_3N_4 Aqueous Suspensions", pp.445-449 in *Ceramic Transactions "Ceramic Processing Science ans Technology"*, Edited by H. Hausner, G.L. Messing, S. Hirano. American Ceramic Society, Westerville, 1995.

[10]A. Salomoni, I. Stamenkovic, A. Tucci and L. Esposito, "Sintering of Alumina and Zirconia Greens Obtained via Slip Casting and Pressure Slip Casting", pp.178-186 in *Ceramic Transactions "Forming Science and Technology for Ceramics"*, Edited by M.J. Cima. American Ceramic Society, Westerville, 1992.

[11]L. Esposito, A. Salomoni, I. Stamenkovic and A. Tucci, "Processing of ZrO_2 - Al_2O_3 Powders: Consolidation and Characterisation of final Products", pp. 37-45 in *Special Meeting on Biomaterials-Rimini 1992,* Edited by I. Stamenkovic, J. Krawcynski. Forschungszentrum, Juelich, 1994.
[12]A. Salomoni, A. Tucci, L. Esposito and I. Stamenkovic, "Forming and Sintering of Multiphase Bioceramics", *Journal of Matererials Science in Medicine,* 5 651-653 (1994).
[13]G. Grathwohl and T. Liu, "Crack Resistance and Fatigue of Transforming Ceramics: I, Materials in the of ZrO_2 - Y_2O_3- Al_2O_3 System", *Journal of the American Ceramic Society* , 74[2] 318-235 (1991).
[14]S.G. Glass and D.J. Green "Mechanical Properties of Infiltrated Alumina -Y-TZP Composites", *Journal of the American Ceramic Society* , 79[9] 2227-2236 (1996).

IN VITRO BIORESORBABLE FIBER DISSOLUTION

S. H. Lee and A. G. Clare
NYS College of Ceramics at Alfred University
2 Pine Street, Alfred, NY 14802

ABSTRACT

To date, there have been many studies, both *in vivo* and *in vitro* on the subject of fiber dissolution. The results obtained from *in vitro* testing are somewhat controversial, since the exact environment experienced by inhaled glass fiber is still a matter of speculation. *In vivo* and *in vitro* studies do not correlate in some cases where apparently durable fiber seems to dissolve rapidly *in vivo*. Small fibers will most often be deposited inside an alveolus[1], and so in order to imitate the *in vivo* conditions more accurately a cellulose ester dialysis membrane was used to simulate the behavior of an alveolar membrane and its effect on glass fiber dissolution. The experiment was also carried out as a function of flow-rate to assess the effect of external flow over the membrane surface on dissolution. Bioresorbable fiber based upon the SiO_2 -Na_2O-K_2O-Al_2O_3-MgO system was studied. The solution was analyzed using Inductively Coupled Plasma spectroscopy (ICP) to show the dissolved species. Tendency of dissolution, and pH change were also measured. The morphology during dissolution, dissolution mechanism, and the flow rate effect are mainly discussed in this paper.

INTRODUCTION

Glass fibers have been used for a number of purposes such as thermal insulation, fiber-reinforced composites, acoustic insulation and synthetic soil for plant growing[2]. The contamination levels of glass fiber in the air have increased about 10 fold since the start of the industrial revolution, to such an extent that glass fiber is present in nearly all ambient air samples regardless of the sampling location (*i.e.* indoors or out)[3]. On average, an adult inhales 10 m^3 of air everyday, and so it is possible that a significant amount of glass fiber is inhaled over the course of a lifetime. Consequently, the biopersistence of glass fiber in the lung is of interest to fiber manufacturers. The biopersistence (chemical durability of fibers in human body) is one of the most important factors, of the so-called 3D's (dose, dimension, and durability). Dose is the quantity of material inhaled over time, dimension means the length, width and aspect ratio of the fibrous material, and durability means the biopersistence of such material in the human lung. A very large dose of a substance, even in the form of very soluble, bioresorbable glass fibers can be toxic, and the risk will decline as the dose declines. It is known that fiber length and diameter are parameters to consider when evaluating carcinogenic potential. Since human bodies have a natural filtration system, large particles or fibers should not infiltrate the lung. Those fibers that are respirable are generally fibers of less than 3 μm in diameter[4]. Short respirable fibers can be cleared by macrophage and/or by the lymphatic system[1]. Long, thin fibers are known to induce the secretion of inflammatory substances by the engulfing macrophage cells. In the long fiber inhalation cases, the duration of fibers in the lung before they are dissolved and/or are cleared is the most important determinant of their toxicity or carcinogenicity.

Fiber dissolution in animal lungs can occur in many environments which differ greatly in corrosivity. The interchange between these environments is poorly understood. Long fibers are most likely to reside in the extracellular matrix, whereas shorter fibers are probably engulfed by macrophages[5-7]. Those fibers which are too long to be fully engulfed by the macrophage will most likely be partially engulfed. Thus, such long fibers will be partially subjected to a near-neutral environment and partially to the acidic environment.

The alveolus is a small, balloon like air sac located at the end of each bronchiole in the lungs. It is lined by a delicate, moist membrane, containing many capillaries which allow for the exchange of respiratory gases[8]. The pH of the surfactant film inside the alveolus is near neutral and the cell liquid inside macrophages has a low pH value so that the dissolution by macrophages can be regarded as corrosion by an acidic solution[9].

In terms of biopersistence, the effect of the alveolar membrane should be considered, since, as mentioned before, the presence of dissolved species around the surface can retard further dissolution and affect the pH and the composition of alveolar surfactant films. In principle, the pH of lung fluid should not radically differ from that of deionized water during dissolution due to the buffer capability of lung fluid[12]. However, it is critical to analyze the elements during dissolution.

The air-blood barrier is composed of the alveolar membrane (epithelium) and pulmonary capillary membrane (endothelium). In addition, The typical pore size were calculated for an alveolar membrane is 8 ~ 20 Å and for a pulmonary capillary membrane is 40 ~ 120 Å[12,13]. The thickness of the air-blood barrier ranges from 0.2μm to 10 μm, and is quite constant for a wide spectrum of mammalian species[8].

Eastes and Hadley[5,6] estimated the "no-disease" limiting k_{dis} which is sensitive to the incidence value that is considered insignificant and the corresponding dose from *in vivo* studies. The average fiber diameter and the fiber density also play a role, although a relatively minor one. The agreement between the dissolution rate constant calculated from the clearance of long fibers *in vivo* and the dissolution rate constant measured *in vitro* provides evidence that the long fibers are being cleared by dissolution. Another possible mechanism for the clearance of the long fibers is the breakage of long fibers into shorter ones that are more readily cleared by macrophages. It is likely that some long fibers are broken, but that the process does not play a significant enough role to explain the results of the RCC (Research and Consulting Company in Geneva, Switzerland) durability study. Yu et al.[7] disputed Eastes' idea that fiber breakage is not the main reason of the long fiber clearance and proposed a new mathematical model of fiber clearance in which the clearance of long fibers is facilitated principally by fiber breakage. Their results showed a strong dependence of the *in vivo* dissolution rate and breakage rate on the *in vitro* dissolution rate, a highly soluble fiber *in vitro* is normally more soluble *in vivo* and easy to break.

The biopersistence of intra-alveolar fibers is an important determinant of their toxicity and carcinogenic potential. Generally, the longer inhaled fibers remain in the alveoli, the more likely they are to impact surrounding tissues. Studies[1,2,10,11,14-18] have shown that the durability and dissolution behavior of fibers in a biological environment depends on their chemical composition, thereby implying that biopersistence is related to glass structure.

In general, the term "chemical durability" is used to describe the resistance of a glass to dissolution by aqueous solutions and atmospheric moisture. As mentioned before, chemical durability is also related to the biopersistence of fiberglass in the human lung. Dissolution of glass fibers in the water is mainly composed of two steps similar to those for bulk glass dissolution, ion exchange and degradation of Si-network structure and further diffusion of water molecules into the glass[19]. Bokasy *et al.*[20] established a theory for dissolution under steady state conditions and applied it to a potash glass, and Doremus[21] developed the interdiffusion model to explain the initial stage of dissolution using a concentration-dependent interdiffusion coefficient. His theory and experimental data were more reasonable than the concentration-independent diffusion coefficient, even though he left the question, "which species replaces the alkali? protons or hydronium ions?" The best evidence for hydronium ions displacing alkali is that there is about 3 for 1 replacement of hydrogen atoms for sodium atoms during the ion exchange process. Nuclear magnetic resonance (NMR) was applied to measure the hydrogen and sodium profiles of hydrated glasses[22]. In that paper, it was experimentally proven that the hydronium ion exchanged rather than proton exchanging, and the Doremus model of interdiffusing ions was extended. More NMR studies have been carried out to show the fact that hydronium ions replace the alkali ion sites in glasses[23,24]. Thus, chemical reaction can be written as:

$$\equiv Si{-}OR_{(gl)} + H_3O^+_{(sol)} \leftrightarrow \equiv Si{-}OH_{(gl)} + H_2O_{(gl)} + R^+_{(sol)} \quad (1)$$

$$\equiv Si{-}O{-}Si\equiv_{(gl)} + OH^-_{(sol)} \leftrightarrow \equiv Si{-}OH_{(gl)} + \equiv Si{-}O^-_{(gl)} \quad (2)$$

Where, equations (1) and (2) respectively show ion exchange and network degradation.

For commercial glasses, it is difficult to specifically describe the dissolution steps such as ion exchange, a silica-rich leached surface layer formation, and fragmentation that occur due to the large number of components present in the glasses. Many *in vitro* studies show that the composition of the fibers can have a strong influence on the dissolution rate[10,17,18]. Potter and Mattson[10,18] provided a thorough summary of compositional effects. Mattson[18] stated that a relationship was found by performing a linear fit of the logarithm of the dissolution rate to the weight percent for glass components. This statistical evaluation implies confounding coefficients of the respective oxide contents, accounting for the different impacts of the individual components. The values of the coefficients depend significantly on the quantity of data used for the analysis and on the type of glass fibers, assuming otherwise constant experimental conditions. Thus, it is not possible to apply a general statistical evaluation to the behavior of soda-lime-silicate glasses, calcium-aluminosilicate or aluminosilicate glasses. However, it is possible to describe some of the physical properties of the glass based upon these empirical coefficients. The durability of the glass is based upon a silica-rich surface layer, and so it can be presumed that the diffusion of the alkali ion through this layer is very difficult, resulting in a surface layer which is resistant to alkaline pH conditions. Thus, this protective layer can play an important role in terms of chemical durability.

German authorities[25] have introduced guidelines (the KI value) with the intent of minimizing commercial availability of biopersistent fibers. These guidelines are based upon an empirical comparison developed during intraperitoneal tests relating the chemical composition of glass fibers to their carcinogenic potency.

$$KI = (c_{Na_2O} + c_{K_2O} + c_{B_2O_3} + c_{CaO} + c_{MgO} + c_{BaO}) - 2\ c_{Al_2O_3} \quad (3)$$

Where, *c*: oxide refers to amount of component in the fiber in wt %
Alumina is known not only to increase the refractoriness of insulation fibers but also to increase the biopersistence[26]. Since the biopersistence is normally proportional to refractoriness, it is hard to optimize the refractoriness and bioresorbability of glass fiber.

Besides the composition of glass fibers, there are many factors that affect biopersistence or chemical durability measurements of a glass in *in vitro* experiments such as surface area, the ratio of surface area of the glass to the volume of the leaching solution ($SA_{(gl)}/V_{(sol)}$) , the frequency of solution replenishment (in the stationary model), temperature, glass composition, thermodynamic stability, and the pH of the solution. The biopersistence of glass fibers is critically dependent on the pH, particularly since many factors end up affecting the pH of the solution. Both the concentration and $SA_{(gl)}/V_{(sol)}$ change with time and so the pH of the attacking solution would also be expected to change correspondingly. Additionally, it is very important to consider the nature of the elements remaining after dissolution. The role of glass fiber's surface is also critical in determining its resistance to dissolution. Bauer[15] studied and reviewed the effect of glass fiber surface on the dissolution rate and breakage in a simulated extracellular lung environment. His results indicate that glass fiber surfaces can show different behavior in body fluid depending upon their initial composition, and the fabrication process conditions. Moreover, the commercial surface coatings are probably not effective in altering the persistence of fibers in such an environment.

Dialysis is a method by which large and small molecules in solution are separated by selective diffusion through a semipermeable membrane. Transfer through the membrane is by diffusion, a process of mass transfer that occurs due to a concentration gradient. There is a molecular screening action by the membrane for solutes of high molecular weight. Although there is never an abrupt cutoff point or critical diameter, there is often a rather sharp decrease of permeability to molecules in a range which is characteristic of the membrane but not of the solute molecules[27]. The molecular weight cut off (MWCO) of the cellulose membrane used here is 100 daltons and the weights of all possible molecules containing dissolved species are, theoretically, under 100 so that they should pass through the membrane. Since the non-electrolyte dialysis membrane method is adapted and no intentional pressure is present, the diffusion through the membrane is mainly caused by a concentration difference on either side of the dialysis membrane. The solvent is water in this study, so imbibition is caused by water and this offers resistance to the diffusion of dissolved species through membrane more than that of a water film of the same physical dimensions. The membrane filled with water molecules will therefore retard diffusion of each species and affect the dissolution of glass fibers.

EXPERIMENTAL PROCEDURE

Sholze[14] pointed out that it is desirable to check all potential variables, if possible, *i.e.* solution's compositional change, weight loss, chemical composition, and morphology of fibers during in vitro experiment. Previous studies clearly show that the composition of fiberglass affects the dissolution rate, and it is related to the morphology during dissolution.

The glass fiber dissolution experiment in a closed system is quite fast and simple to perform, enabling many samples to be investigated. The results, though, are not realistic, as the dissolution of the fibers alters the composition and the pH of the solution during the experiment. Thus, the experimental time period should be short.

In this study bioresorbable glass fibers (biofibers) that are designed to dissolve away faster when they are inhaled and deposited into alveoli were used. The average diameter (8.6 μm) was calculated from BET data, assuming that the fibers are continuously cylindrical. Scanning Electron Microscopy (SEM) images of the as-received fibers were taken to inspect the surface, since the dissolution behavior can be altered due to the aging effect of moisture in the atmosphere. The fibers had clean surfaces, but they were long and tangled. To imitate the airborne fibers and increase the surface area, they were chopped using a mortar and pestle to achieve a uniform surface area, 0.32 m^2/g.

1 g of sample fibers were used for the experiment. For the dialysis membrane-free method (DMF), sample fibers were put into deionized (DI) water and dispersed by a shaking bath. The temperature was maintained at 36.5 °C and the sample bottles were agitated at a frequency of 60 oscillations/min. For the dialysis membrane method, a membrane tube (1×7 cm) was filled with chopped fibers and put into the DI water.

For the free fiber, non-dialysis method, after dissolution, after various time period (usually 7, 14, 21, and 28 days), the solution was filtered through a membrane filter whose pore size was 4.5 μm to remove the remaining tiny fragments of glass fibers. The filtrated solution was analyzed using Inductively Coupled Plasma emission spectroscopy (ICP). pH was also measured. The residual glass fibers remaining on the filter were dried in the oven for 10 hours at 110°C and weighed.

For the dialysis membrane method (DM), the external solution was similarly analyzed, although filtration was not required. The internal solution was also supposed to be analyzed, but, since there were many tiny fragments and the amount of liquid was too small to be filtered, the inside solution was unable to be analyzed. The membrane effect upon the dissolution rate can be partially understood by comparing the dialysis membrane method with the non-dialysis membrane method. Surface morphologies were investigated by SEM, and Energy Dispersive X-ray spectroscopy (EDX). All experiments were repeated more than twice.

The infinite dilute system (flowing model) experiments were carried out to compensate for disadvantages of closed system (stationary model) experiments. The advantage of the infinitely dilute system is that conditions can be kept constant, and a constant dissolution rate can be established over a longer period. The disadvantages are that the method is time consuming and demands more resources (individual pumps, *etc.*). The results are dependent on the flow rate, so absolute values cannot be obtained as the flow rate of liquid in the lung cannot be determined. Perturbation of the fluid surrounding inhaled fibers is expected to be small, and, therefore, dissolution fluid flowing continuously over a few fibers would be a good flowing system.

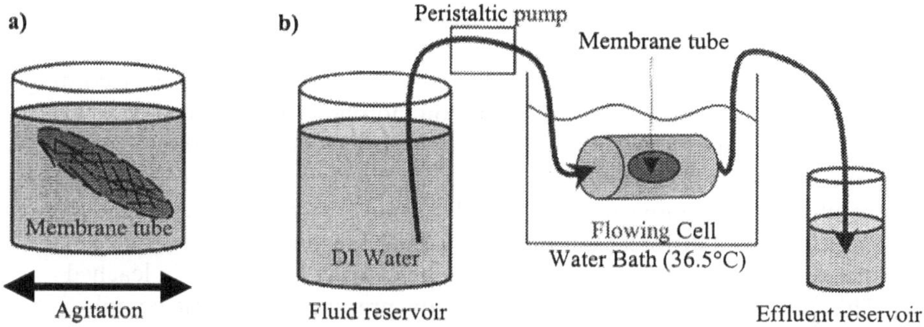

Figures I. Experimental arrangements for the dialysis membrane method a) Static and b) Infinitely dilute system

The membrane filter whose pore diameter is 0.4 μm was used for both inlet and outlet of the flow cell in the non-dialysis membrane method. This pore size was determined by previous conventional *in vitro* studies[10,16,18] which indicate that 0.4 μm is small enough. 1g of fibers was weighed and put in the flow cells, or placed into the membrane tube. DI water flowed over the sample fibers or the dialysis membrane tube through the flow cells, and the effluent was collected after 7, 14, 21, and 28 days. The collected solution was analyzed by ICP, and pH was also measured. The surface morphology was inspected as well.

In previous studies, the flow rate was approximately 100 ml/day on average, but could be in the range of 50 to 200 ml/day, if artificial lung fluid was used. In this study, deionized water (pH ~ 6.8) was used instead of artificial lung fluid such as Gamble solution, since the main purpose of this study was to analyze the dissolved species in solution and characterize the effect of the dialysis membrane. Thus, the flow rate should be faster to avoid a large pH change during dissolution. The dissolution product concentration in solution may approach saturation values, slowing the dissolution or changing its nature. Therefore, flow rate affects the dissolution rate and the morphology. The infinitely dilute system experiment was performed as a function of flow rate (1000 ml/wk, 2000 ml/wk, and 3000 ml/wk).

RESULTS AND DISCUSSION

Morphology and Dissolution Mechanism

If glass fibers are brought in contact with a solution of near-neutral pH, alkali ions will be extracted into the solution in preference to silica and an alkali-depleted layer is formed on the surface of the virgin fibers[14,19-21,28-32]. It is known that the formation of this Si-rich layer retards further dissolution by protecting the fiber from leaching[18]. The thickness and the compactness of the Si-rich layer can vary with the composition of the glass fibers and the attacking solution.

The morphology during glass fiber dissolution has been studied according to the composition of glass fiber[10]. Dissolution morphology has been observed to change as a function of dissolution rate using the rod of glass. Neither the cause nor the mechanism was explained, but it was argued that the change that retards the dissolution of the more soluble glasses has been identified. Fibers recovered from animals show a different morphology from those generated by *in vitro* experiments. There was a reduction in diameter with no evidence of a leached layer. This fact might be attributed to the *in vivo* presence of organic complexing agents, which remove the leached material as it is formed. Its mechanical weakness may lead to physical removal while in the animal or during the extraction process. The absence of the leached layer *in vivo* suggests that the leaching process is the rate-determining step *in vivo* as it is in *in vitro* studies.

The calculated KI value of the biofiber reported here is 41 and it is known that a KI value of ≥ 40 will lead to the ultimate dissolution of the sample fibers[25]. Figure II shows the SEM image of it's peeling behavior. This kind of morphology was not observed in the standard fibers' dissolution. It was already stated that the silica rich layer was formed because of an ion exchange process. When H_3O^+ replaces Na^+ in the glass fibers' surface, swelling takes place. This swelling can be mainly attributed to the volume difference between ions that participate in the ion exchange process. The H_3O^+ ion (~0.132 Å) is bigger than the sodium ion (0.98 Å). When the large ions exchange sites with smaller alkali ions in glass, provided the temperature is lower than the glass transition temperature, then the large ions will be squeezed into smaller spaces, generating a surface compression[33]. Inversely, beneath the ion exchanged surface layer, tensile stress will develop. The gap between compression and tensile stress can be the driving force to break apart the surface layer from the core. Therefore, ion stuffing occurred during ion exchange so that a stress was applied to the ion-exchanged region (surface). When the stress was big enough to separate the surface layer from the core of the fiber, the peeling behavior manifested.

It is known that the surface layer before peeling plays the role of a protective layer against attack by the solution[10,34]. The EDX data (Figure II) clearly show that the surface layer is depleted of sodium while the core of the fiber retains the initial sodium content. Of course, there is no sodium in the chips from the fibers that are the fragments of the surface layer. These fragments can be cleared by macrophages in human lung quite easily. Subsequently, it is natural that the fracture of the outer protective layers can accelerate the clearance.

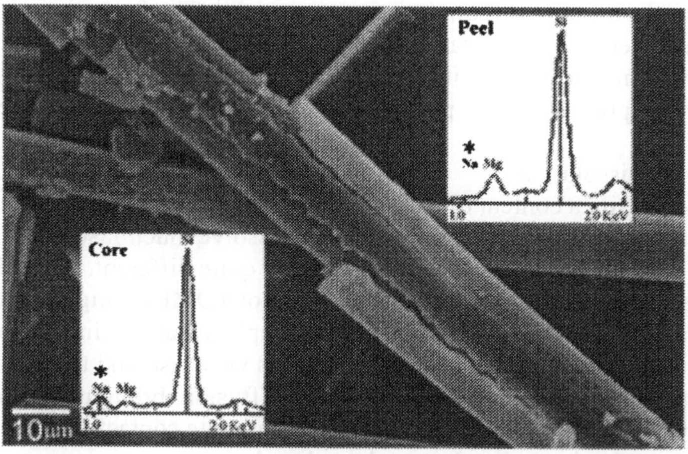

Figure II. Peeling behavior (SEM image and EDX data in white boxes)

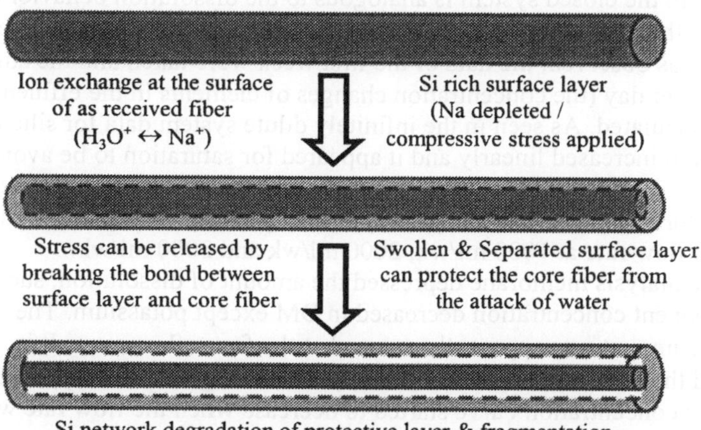

Figure III. Scheme of bioresorbable fiber dissolution

The ion exchanged, sodium depleted, and silica-rich surface layer will be mechanically weak. The interdiffusion through modifier channels in the random network model, rather than through the network regions, would lead to structural defects composed of sections of modifier channels that are filled with water. Such defects will intersect the glass surface and hydrogen bonds across the defects are significantly weaker than ionic bonding. These bonds can play the role of a "Griffith's flaw" and be easily broken by physical agitation (by macrophages or by swelling and shrinking alveoli during respiration)[35]. The formation of the protective layer seems to be negative in terms of bioresorbability, but its mechanical weakness can make it possible for the separated surface layer to be cleared by macrophages or even physical agitation by alveolar membrane.

Flow Effect on Dissolution

Since the silica content of the biofibers is much lower than that in regular fiber, the network structure is very loose. They dissolve much faster than standard insulation fibers and the dissolution mechanism is quite different. The pH change during the test in the dialysis membrane free method (DMF) is bigger than that in the dialysis membrane method (DM). This fact implies that the dissolution process of biofibers (both DM and NDF) proceeds very fast, and they immediately reach the critical concentration for diffusion through the membrane to start. However, more dissolved species are in intimate contact with the fibers in DM so that they also immediately retard the dissolution.

The membrane depresses the dissolution of bioresorbable fiber probably because it retards the fragmentation of the protective surface layer. The dissolution in the closed system is analogous to the dissolution behavior of biofibers in the infinitely dilute system where the flow-rate is zero. Since saturation was observed, the data of the first week were taken and the amount of dissolution per day (the concentration changes of elements in the effluents per a day) was calculated. As seen in the infinitely dilute system data for silicon, the concentration increased linearly and it appeared for saturation to be avoided successfully. The increases of Si, Na, K, Ca concentration per day were also calculated for each flow rate and plotted. The experiment was performed as a function of flow rate at 1000 ml/wk, 2000 ml/wk and 3000 ml/wk.

The dialysis membrane depressed the amount of dissolution, such that each component concentration decreased in DM except potassium. The dissolution amount was apparently reduced at the faster flow rates. It is recognized that the faster the flow rate is, the less the glass fiber dissolved. The slope of the concentration curve started to decrease when the flow rate was sufficiently large to become a contributing factor. The decrease was sensitive within a certain flow rate range. However, above or below it, the slope was not a strong function of flow rate changes. This could explain why the slope decreased very much from that at 1000 ml/wk, whereas the slope at 2000 ml/wk and that at 3000 ml/wk are almost the same within the error bars.

When the flow-rate was sufficiently low, the leaching or dissolution of alkalis consumed hydronium ions in the DI water and it raised the pH. Moreover, the dissolution product concentrations in solution approached saturation values and affected (slowed down) the dissolution.

These effects led to variable and unpredictable changes in dissolution rate. Mattson[17] showed that the dissolution rate can increase or decrease by small amounts for most glass fiber compositions and can decrease by large amounts for some rapidly dissolving glasses when simulated lung fluid is used. There was considerable variation both in the magnitude of the measured rates and in the relative ranking of the different compositions in terms of rate.

In the case of the dialysis membrane method, the dissolution mechanism were more complicated. The attacking agents, *i.e.* hydronium, and hydroxyl ions, should permeate through the membrane and the dissolved species also should permeate through the membrane to be cleared away. This counter-diffusion through the barrier (membrane) can imitate that which occurs through the real alveolar membrane.

In the biofiber dissolution, the decrease of dissolution rate as the flow-rate increased implies that attacking agents just got swept away by the flow rate before they have a chance to actually react. Thus, H_3O^+ and OH^- ions just pass away rather than attack the glass surface when the flow-rate is sufficiently high. However, this might not be an explanation for the dissolution in the simulated lung fluid because Mattson[17] also showed that the dissolution rate could increase as flow rate gets faster when the simulated lung fluid is used. Since diverse alkalis exist in the solution, the mechanisms would be more complicated.

Figures IV show the flow rate effect on the changes of pH and concentrations of dissolved species. Both in DM and DMF, concentrations became independent of flow rate between 1000 ml/week and 2000 ml/week. The average pH change in DM became independent of flow rate when it was over 2000 ml/week and in DMF became constant at flow rate of over 1000 ml/week. The concentration of silicon was the most sensitive to the flow rate and usually decreased by the biggest factor as flow rate increased. The amount of sodium in the effluent also decreased in the infinitely dilute system. These indicate that both the leaching process and network degradation are much slower in the infinitely dilute system and that network degradation can be retarded more in the infinitely dilute system under this experimental condition. The comparison of concentration change curves between DM and DMF shows that the dissolution in DM was depressed. It is recognized in this study that the concentration of potassium is almost constant at any flow rate and there is no significant difference between DM and DMF.

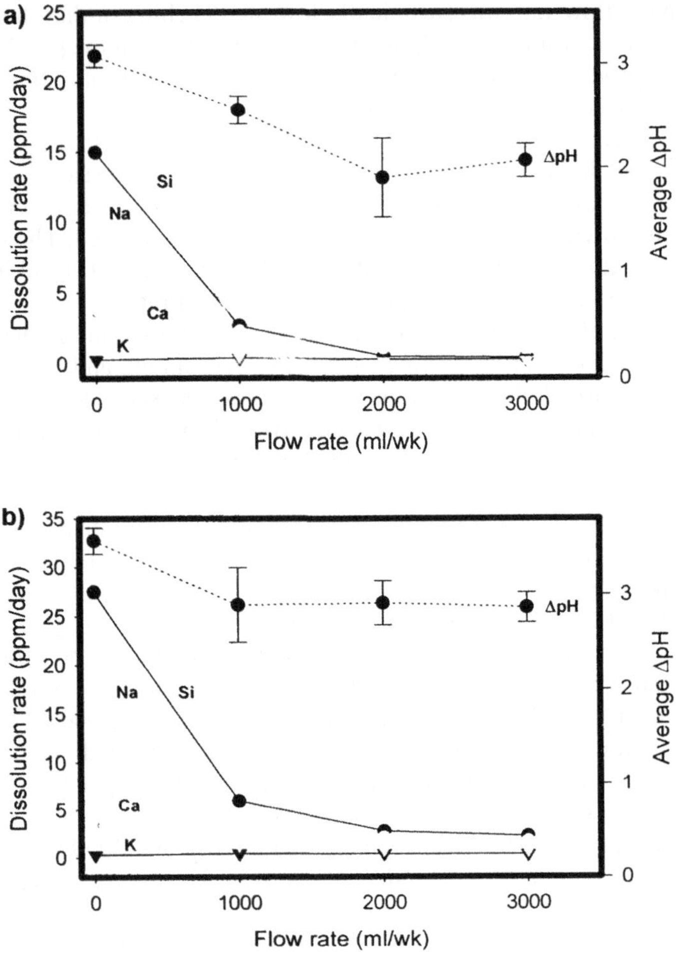

Figure IV. Flow rate effect on the bioresorbable fiber dissolution
a) Dialysis membrane method, b) Dialysis membrane-free method

CONCLUSION

The dialysis membrane method was adapted to simulate the environment of inhaled and deposited fibers and showed this can be effective and definitely affected the dissolution rate. There have been many studies to determine which glass fibers are more bioresorbable or biocompatible using the conventional *in vitro* and *in vivo* methods. However, the *in vitro* dialysis membrane method is strongly recommended for a more realistic *in vitro* environment because the inhaled fibers will be mostly trapped and deposited in the surfactant film inside the alveolar membrane[1].

During dissolution, the peeling behavior was observed showing that the formation of sodium depleted surface layer separated from the unaltered core where sodium ions are retained. The ion exchange process followed by stress development due to the volume difference can explain this fact. The formation of a mechanically weak surface layer can have a positive effect in terms of bioresorbability.

The flow rate effect on biofiber dissolution was also studied. The amount of dissolved species in the effluents decrease as flow rate increases. Between 1000 ml/week and 2000 ml/week, they become independent of the flow rate and the concentration of silicon is the most sensitive to the flow rate. The average change of pH during dissolution also decreases as flow rate increases.

REFERENCES

[1]P. Gross and D. C. Braun, *Toxic and Biomedical Effects of Fibers,* Noyers Publications, New Jersey, 1984.

[2]J. Caceres, J. E. Garcia-Hernandez, P. Callejas and J. M. Rincon, "Microstructural and Analytical Characterisation of Some Commercial and Experimental Mineral Glass Fibres," *Glass Technology*, 34 [4] 159-162 (1993).

[3]J. A. Hoskins, R. C. Brown and I. C. Alexander, "Biological Persistence of Mineral Fibres found as Contaminants of Indoor Air," *Environ. Tech.*, 13, 361-366 (1992).

[4]J. G. Hadley, "Health Aspects of Fibrous Glass: Current Status," *Ceram. Eng. Sci. Proc.*, 14 [3-4] 181-189.

[5]W. Eastes and J. G. Hadley, "A Mathematical Model of Fiber Carcinogenicity and Fibrosis in Inhalation and Intraperitoneal Experiments in Rats," *Inhalation Toxicol.*, 8, 323-343 (1996).

[6]W. Eastes and J. G. Hadley, "Dissolution of Fibers Inhaled by Rats," *Inhalation Toxicol.*, 7, 179-196 (1995).

[7]C. P. Yu, Y. T. Dai, P. M. Boymel, B. K. Zoitos, G. Oberdoster and M. J. Utell, "Fiber Clearance Model in Rats," *Inhalation Toxicol.*, 10, 253-274 (1998).

[8]E. R. Weibel, "The Ultrastructure of the Alveolar-Capillary Membrane or Barrier"; pp. 9-27 in *The Pulmonary Circulation and Interstitial Stace.* edited by F. A. Hecht. The University of Chicago Press, Illinois, 1969.

[9]I. Carr, *A Review of Ultrastructure and Function,* Academic Press, New York, 1973 .

[10]R. M. Potter and S. M. Mattson, "Glass Fiber Dissolution in a Physiological Saline Solution," *Glastech. Ber*, 64 [Nr. 1] 16-28 (1991).

[11]V. R. Christensen, S. Lund Jensen, M. Guldberg and O. Kamstrup, "Effect of pH and Chemical Composition of MMVF on Dissolution," *Environ. Health Perspect.*, 102 [5] 83-86 (1994).

[12]G. M. Kanapilly, "Alvolar Microenvironment and Its Relationship to the Retention and Transport into Blood of Aerosols Deposited in the Alveoli," *Health Phys.,* 32 [2] 99-100 (1977).

[13]A. E. Taylor and K. A. Gaar Jr., "Estimation of Equivalent Pore Radii of Pulmonary Capillary and Alveolar Membranes," *Am. J. Physiol.*, 218 [4] 1133-1140 (1970).

[14]H. Scholze, "Durability Investigations on Siliceous Man-Made Mineral Fibers A Critical Review," *Glasstech. Ber.*, 61 [Nr. 6] 161-171 (1988).

[15]J. F. Bauer, "Interaction of Glass Fiber with Physiological Fluids: The Role of Surface", in *XVIII International Congress on Glass.* Edited by M. K. Choudhary, N. T. Huff and C. H. Drummond III. San Francisco, California,1998.

[16]M. Guldberg, V. R. Christensen, W. Krois and K. Sebastian, "Method for Determining In-Vitro Dissolution Rates of Man-Made Vitreous Fibres," *Glastech. Ber.*, 68 [6] 181-187 (1995).

[17]S. M. Mattson, "Glass Fiber Dissolution in Simulated Lung Fluid and Measures Needed to Improve Consistency and Correspondence to *In Vivo* Dissolution," *Environ. Health Perspect.*, 102 [Suppl. 5] 87-90 (1994).

[18]S. M. Mattson, "Glass Fibres in Simulated Lung Fluid: Dissolution Behaviour and Analytical Reqiurements," *Ann. Occup. Hyg*, 38 [6] 857-877 (1994).

[19]A. Paul, "Chemical Durability of Glasses; a Thermodynamic Approach," *J. Mater. Sci.*, 12**,** 2246-2268 (1977).

[20]Z. Bokasy, G. Bouquet and S. Dobos, "Diffusion Processes in the Surface Layer of Glass," *Phys. Chem. Glasses*, 8 [4] 140-144 (1967).

[21]R. H. Doremus, "Interdiffusion of Hydrogen and Alkali Ions in a Glass Surface," *J. Non-Cryst. Solids*, 19**,** 137-144 (1975).

[22]W. A. Lanford, K. Davis, P. Lamarche, T. Laursen, R. Groleau and R. H. Doremus, "Hydration of Soda-Lime Glass," *J. Non-Cryst. Solids*, 33**,** 249-266 (1979).

[23]I. S. T. Tsong, C. A. Houser, W. B. White, A. L. Wintenberg, P. D. Miller and C. D. Moak, "Evidence for Interdiffusion of Hydronium and Alkali Ions in Leached Glasses," *Appl. Phys. Lett.*, 39 [8] 669-670 (1981).

[24]L. R. Pederson, D. R. Baer, G. L. McVay, K. F. Ferris and M. H. Engelhard, "Reaction of Silicate Glasses in Water Labelled with D and ^{18}O," *Phys. Chem. Glasses*, 31 [5] (1990).

[25]"Technical Rules for Hazardous Materials" *Verzeichnis Krebserzeugender, Erbgutverandernder oder Fortphlanzungsgefahrdender Stoffe,* Technishe Regeln Fur Gefahrstoffe, 1994.

[26]I. C. Alexander and G. A. Jubb, "Develoment of a Soluble High-Temperate Insulation Fiber," *Glass Sci. Technol.*, 70 [12] (1997).

[27]S. B. Tuwiner, L. P. Miller and W. E. Brown, *Diffusion and Membrane Technology,* Reinhold Publishing Corporation, New York, 1962 .

[28]C. G. Pantano, "Glass Surfaces," *Rev. of Solid State Sci.*, 3, 379-408 (1989).

[29]C. V. Gokularathnam, R. W. Gould and L. L. Hench, "Effect of "Water" on the Structure of Vitreous Silica," *Phys. Chem. Glasses*, 16 [2] 13-16 (1975).

[30]H. Scholze, "Glass-Water Interactions," *J. Non-Cryst. Solids*, 102, 1-10 (1988).

[31]J. B. Donnet, R. Batistella and B. Chatenet, "A Study of the Surface of Glass Fibres," *Glass Technol.*, 16 [6] 139-148 (1975).

[32]J. Schafer and H. A. Schaeffer, "Leaching of Alkali Silicate Glasses - Formation of Hydrated Layers, Surface-and Diffusion-Controlled Kinetics," *Riv. Stu. Sper. Vetro*, [5] 79-82 (1984).

[33]A. K. Varshneya, *Fundamentals of Inorganic Glasses,* Academic Press, New York, 1994 .

[34]L. L. Hench, "Glass Corrosion and Durability," *J. Non-Cryst. Solids*, 19, 27-39 (1975).

[35]R. J. Hand, and A. B. Seddon, "An Hypothesis on the Nature of Griffith's Cracks in Alkali Silicate and Silica Glasses," *Phys. Chem. Glasses*, 38 [1] 11-14 (1997).

L. R. Pederson, D. R. Baer, G. L. McVay, K. F. Ferris and M. H. Engelhard, [illegible]

[illegible]

SCOPE OF PIEZOELECTRIC DEVICES IN DETERMINING INNER EAR FUNCTION

N. Mukherjee and R. D. Roseman
Dept. of Materials Science and Engineering
University of Cincinnati
Cincinnati, OH 45221-0012.

J. P. Willging,
Dept. of Otolaryngology, Head, and Neck Surgery
University of Cincinnati
Cincinnati, OH 45267-0528.

ABSTRACT

A better understanding of the fundamental phenomena occurring in both the healthy and the artificially stimulated cochlea will greatly aid in the engineering of more effective cochlear implant devices and will enhance mankind's knowledge of inner ear function. This investigation was conducted to probe the feasibility of use of specially developed piezoelectric sensors to shed light on these phenomena. An external mechanical model of the cochlea has been fabricated and suitable piezoelectric devices tested. Results from initial experiments aimed at device development, investigation of cochlear acoustics *in vitro*, and the feasibility of a piezoelectric cochlear implant are presented. It is shown that piezoelectric devices offer a novel and extremely useful means of not only investigating cochlear acoustics, but also of the possible development of a novel piezoelectric cochlear implant.

INTRODUCTION

The mammalian inner ear cochlea has been a subject of scientific attention over the past several decades. Efforts have concentrated on one hand on understanding the basic acoustical, physiological, biophysical, and neural phenomena[1-14] which work in harmony to make the cochlea one of the most sensitive and complex systems known, and on the other hand, in the development and use of cochlear implant devices for implantation in patients suffering from sensorineural hearing loss.[15-21] Extensive theoretical studies have attempted to explain inner ear mechanisms.[2,10-14] Experimental investigations of intracochlear acoustical phenomena have been rare because of the practical difficulties involved.[7-9] These difficulties also limit the range and extent of *in vivo* experimentation. Though a lot has been uncovered regarding cochlear function, a clear picture has not yet emerged. Similarly, although cochlear implants are now employed, several questions regarding their functioning remain unanswered.[17]

The present study aims to develop special piezoelectric sensors for: 1) *in vitro* and *in vivo* characterization of cochlear acoustics; and, 2) development of a possible piezoelectric cochlear implant. The use of piezoelectrics in the attempt to overcome hearing disorders is not new. Piezoelectrics have been used in middle ear implants, in which the middle ear bones are vibrated by an external coil-battery-amplifier-piezoelectric vibrator setup.[22] The development and use of piezoelectric devices for the above-mentioned applications has, however, not been reported.

MATERIALS CHALLENGES

A piezoelectric based pressure measurement system was used by Nedzelnitsky to measure intracochlear acoustical phenomena.[7] In general, a piezoelectric *in vivo/in vitro* cochlear pressure measurement device must overcome the following challenges: 1) Dimensional restrictions imposed on the device. Not only does the device have to be small enough to fit in the cochlear scalae, it has to be small enough to prevent 'loading' effects; 2) Decreased piezoelectric hydrostatic stress and voltage coefficients (d_h and g_h); and, 3) Acoustic impedance mismatch with water.

Piezoelectric Cochlear Implant

Consideration for use of piezoelectric devices[23] stems from the facts that: a) Piezoelectrics are used routinely in applications that involve detection of human voice, musical notes, etc., demonstrating the ability to transduce complex acoustic stimuli[24-26]; b) Being natural transducers, piezoelectrics function without the need for an external power supply, presenting the possibility of obtaining an entirely 'stand-alone' unit; c) Such a device will provide, at once, a *bipolar* electrode arrangement[18]; and, d) Such a device would be non-invasive to the cochlea once implanted. Indeed, the successful working of the device would necessitate proper mechanical functioning of the cochlea. Such an implant could be used purely as a research device, to provide a better understanding, by means of experiments both *in vivo* and *in vitro*, of both cochlear phenomena and cochlear implant functioning.

Fabrication of a piezoelectric cochlear implant is a challenging task: not only does the transducer have to detect the mechanical pressures, the sensitivity of the device must be adequate so that the generated charge is sufficient to stimulate surviving nerve fibers in the cochlea, without any need for amplification. Piezoelectric transducers are used widely under hydrostatic conditions, but the effective piezoelectric stress (d_h) and voltage (g_h) coefficients under these conditions are notoriously low. This is especially the case for lead zirconate-titanate (PZT) and barium titanate ceramic materials.[27] Fabrication of piezoelectric ceramic/polymer composites has vastly improved the hydrostatic coefficients: improvements of greater than an order of magnitude have been achieved by using a PZT/foamed polyurethane composite.[28] Also, the polymer piezoelectric polyvinylidene fluoride (PVDF) is much more flexible than ceramic piezoelectrics and can easily be formed as very thin films.[26,29,30] These materials are likely candidates for the fabrication of a piezoelectric cochlear implant.

Another disadvantage of using ceramic piezoelectrics underwater (the cochlear fluid, perilymph, is a saline solution) is the large acoustic impedance mismatch between water and ceramic, leading to decreased transduction efficiency of the piezoelectric.[31] Quarter wavelength thick impedance matching layers can minimize this mismatch,[32] but for audio frequencies, the thicknesses of such layers are significant. The problem is much less when PVDF is used, since the acoustic impedance of PVDF is not significantly larger than that of water.[30]

Matters are further complicated by the dimensional restrictions imposed on the device. Not only does the device have to be small enough to fit into the cochlear ducts, it has to be small enough to prevent any substantial loading effects. The cochlea cannot accommodate a device larger than ~ 1.5mm x 1.5mm x 1mm if the device is placed across the transverse cross-section. On the other hand, if placed along the length of the scala tympani, the device can be several millimeters long. It has to, however, be flexible to be able to fit into the curving cochlea. Not only are such small devices difficult to fabricate, a lower surface area will lower the total charge produced and necessitate a commensurate increase in sensitivity. The following calculation determines the charge that will be generated by a piezoelectric device made of the best PZT/foamed polyurethane composite[28] when a pressure of 120 dB SPL is applied. The figure of 120 dB SPL is chosen as a high value of pressures present in the cochlea.[7,8] It should be mentioned here that the perilymph fluid in the cochlea is electrically conducting with a resistivity of ~ 70 ohm-cm.[33] Under such conditions, the piezoelectric can be considered to be in an *electrically free* environment.[24,34,35] The use of free piezoelectric ($d_h = 225 \times 10^{-12}$ CN^{-1})[29] and dielectric ($\varepsilon_r = 40$)[29] constants in making calculations are thus justified. Using these values and for a device of dimensions 1mm x 1mm x 0.1mm and a pressure of 120 dB SPL, which corresponds to 20 Pascals (ref. 20 μPa), the charge on the surface of the device is approximately 4.5×10^{-15} C.

This calculation is in a sense ideal, in that it assumes complete impedance matching between the fluid medium and the piezoelectric, there being no question of impedance match/mismatch in contact stress/strain measurements of piezoelectric constants.

Figure 1 is a plot showing the expected charge that will be produced by present day engineering piezoelectric materials,[28,29,36] over a sound pressure range of 80-180 dB SPL. A constant device dimension of 1mm x 1mm x 0.1mm has been assumed. Cochlear implants are described in terms of nanocoulombs of charge per cycle of stimulation.[37] To facilitate comparison with present day cochlear implants, the value of the peak charge produced by a piezoelectric device during the cycle (i.e., at maximum strain) has been plotted against the sound pressure level present in Figure 1. It has been stated that the threshold value of nervous stimulation for modiolar electrodes (direct contact with the nerves) is ~ 5 nC/cycle of pulsatile stimulation, and for scala tympani electrodes it is approxim-

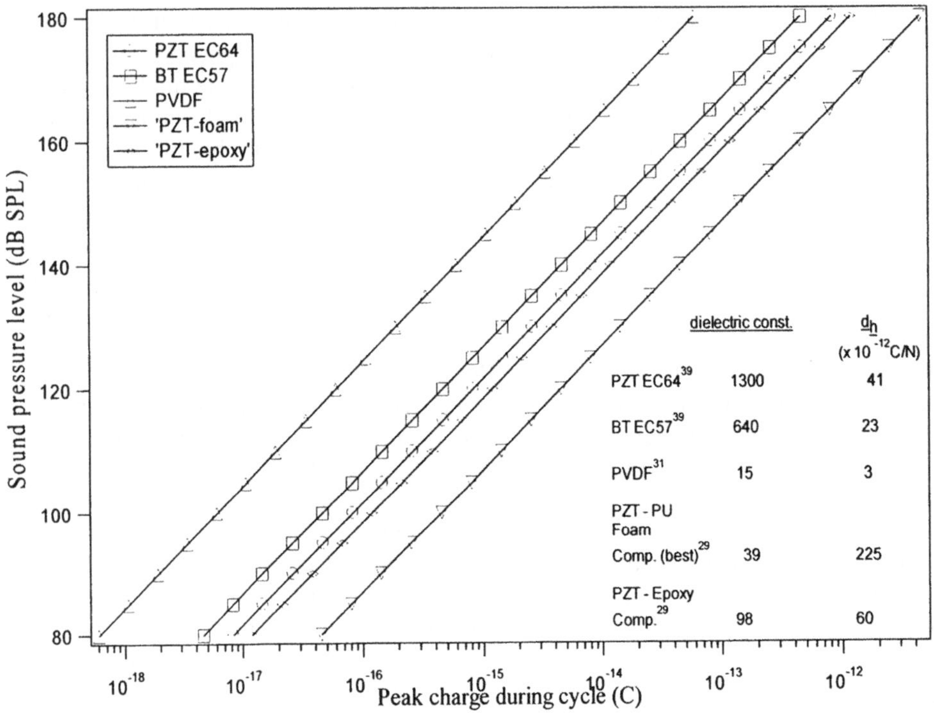

Figure 1. Plot showing the expected charge developed by modern piezoelectric materials in the pressure range of 80-180 dB SPL. Plots generated from data in the inset table.

-ately twice this value.[37] From Figure 1 it is clear that none of the materials are capable of producing charge of this magnitude.

Thus, it is initially evident that the development of a successful piezoelectric cochlear implant is a challenging task indeed, if not nearly impossible with the present state of the art. Not only does it require fabrication of very small piezoelectric devices; it also demands an increase in sensitivity of even the best materials by several orders of magnitude. However, the cochlear environment is far from simple and, in general, not well understood. These issues, along with recent *in vivo* results which are contrary to theoretical predictions, are discussed in detail in a previous paper. Moreover, *in vitro* data presented subsequently are also in contrast to theory. All these observations lead to the conclusion that it would be premature to rule out the possibility of a piezoelectric cochlear implant solely on the basis of theoretical calculations.

EXPERIMENTATION

External Test Station

The goal was the design and development of an external mechanical analogue of the cochlea in order to devise a means of testing suitable piezoelectric materials. An illustration of the mechanisms of acoustic wave generation and propagation in the cochlea is depicted in the simple schematic diagram of Figure 2, which is a functional representation of the cochlea.[3,4] From Figure 2 it can be

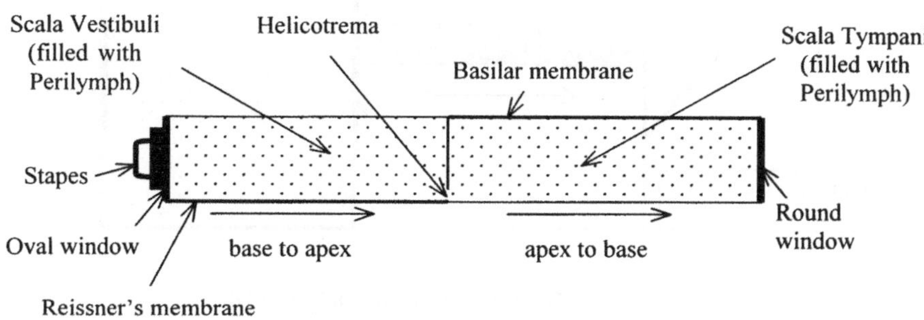

Figure 2. Schematic illustration of mechanical functions of the cochlea.

seen that the pressure is transferred to the oval window diaphragm by the stapes and travels through the Perilymph of the scala vestibuli all the way to the apical turn. At the apical turn, the pressure wave enters the scala tympani through the small opening, the helicotrema, and travels down to the basal turn through the scala tympani. The round window diaphragm acts as a pressure release window, enabling the excess pressure to be released into the middle ear air cavity.[3] The external test cell was modeled on this simple concept. Figure 3 shows a schematic diagram of the test cell and the pressure generation unit. The end of the piston was capped with a flat circular aluminum disc. For the purposes of testing, the piston was positioned against the front rubber diaphragm and the speaker was powered.* The power to the speaker and the amplitude and frequency of vibration were controlled by means of a function generator. The cell was filled with 18 Mohm deionized water and all experiments were carried out at room temperature. All piezoelectric devices tested were coated with an insulating layer of rubber, thus making the device performance insensitive to the solution salinity. Deionized water was used for the sake of maintaining a standard. The working principle of this setup is thus a *mechanical* analogue of the actual mechanism in the ear shown in Figure 2. The test cell and the pressure generation system were placed inside a Faraday cage.

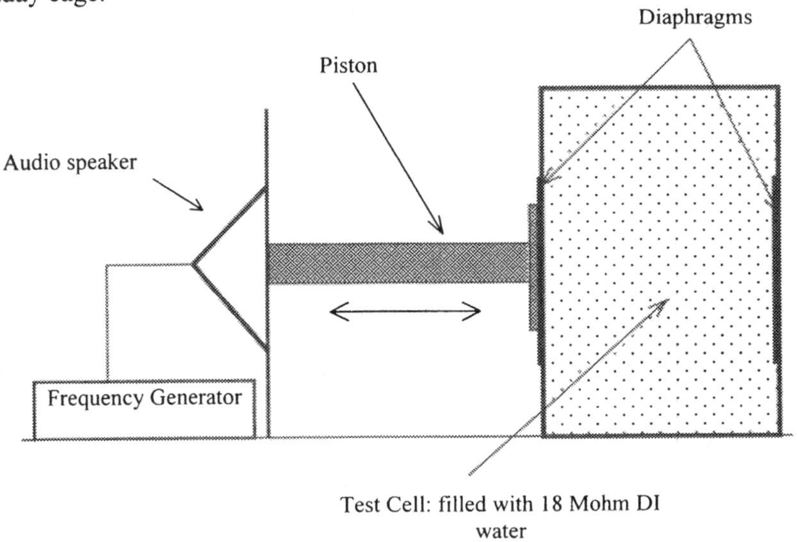

Figure 3. Schematic of test cell and pressure generation system.

Experiments were conducted on ceramic samples to which wires were attached on each of the two electrodes. The voltage generated across the electrodes when the samples were subjected to the acoustic pressure in the test

* Throughout this paper, "front diaphragm" will be used to refer to the diaphragm at which the pressure is transferred from the pressure generation system to the fluid within the test cell. This diaphragm is, then, analogous to the Oval window of the cochlea. The term "rear diaphragm" will be used to refer to the diaphragm on the opposite wall of the cell. This diaphragm is analogous to the Round window.

cell was detected by a data acquisition system via an unity gain operational amplifier. The data acquisition system used was a Wavebook/512™ (IOTech, Inc., Oh, USA) equipped with a WBK14 dynamic signal conditioning module. The hardware units were controlled automatically from a computer loaded with support software.

Preparation of Device for *In Vitro* Tests

It is well known that PZT compositions, in general, exhibit better piezoelectric properties compared to $BaTiO_3$ compositions.[24] PZT compositions, however, incorporate substantial concentrations of the toxic metal lead (Pb), as such, their implantation into the human body should be avoided. An ongoing effort, therefore, also employed fabrication of piezoelectric devices with substantially good properties from $BaTiO_3$ compositions. Table I lists the dielectric and piezoelectric data of the high quality ceramics used. However, since the PZT ceramics possess better piezoelectric properties, results presented here focus on these materials.

PZT devices of the following dimensions and electrodes were prepared for experiments: 1) 5mm x 5mm x 0.260mm with 25μm thick Ag electrodes; 2) 2mm x 1mm x 0.260mm with 25μm thick Ag electrodes. For the purposes of testing, glass coated copper (Cu) wires, of diameter 150μm, were attached to both electrodes of the samples. One end of the wires were attached to the Ag electrodes by means of conducting Ag paste and the other end to the input of the data acquisition system by means of a low noise BNC cable. In order to overcome detection problems associated with immersion in a fluid, the wire-attached PZT samples were coated with a dielectric layer of Neoprene rubber (Aldrich Chem. Co., WI, USA), in an effort to duplicate commercial underwater piezoelectric devices, which are usually enclosed in a Neoprene sheath. The rubber solution was made by dissolving 10 wt.% Neoprene in Toluene ($C_6H_5CH_3$) (Fisher Scientific, Inc., NJ, USA). Piezoelectrics were coated with Neoprene by means of spin coating and dip coating.

Table I. Dielectric and piezoelectric properties of the ceramic compositions used.

Material	ε_r (@ 1 kHz)	d_{33} (x 10^{-12} M/V)	g_{33} (x 10^{-3} V-M/N)	k_{33}
BT	1540	150	11.0	0.38
PZT1	1050	220	23.7	0.62
PZT2	3450	583	19.1	0.75

RESULTS AND DISCUSSION

Calibration of Test Cell

Before experiments with actual piezoelectric devices were started, it was necessary to calibrate the sound pressure levels (SPL) obtained in the test cell fluid by means of a hydrophone of known sensitivity. For this purpose, a PCMH-2™ hydrophone, manufactured by EDO Corporation, UT, USA, was used. The PCMH-2 was lowered into the fluid (18 Mohm de-ionized water) of the test cell. The hydrophone's position was kept constant near the center of the test cell for calibration. Figure 4 shows the calibration curve. It can be seen that the maximum sound pressure level obtained was ~ 140 dB SPL at 100Hz. The pressure dropped sharply at 200Hz and then remained more or less constant in the range 115-125 dB SPL up to 600Hz, after which there was another sudden drop to ~85 dB SPL at 800Hz. The sound pressure measured at 1KHz was ~ 87 dB SPL. Normal conversational speech generates pressures of 50-75 dB SPL and intracochlear fluid pressures reach up to ~120 dB SPL.

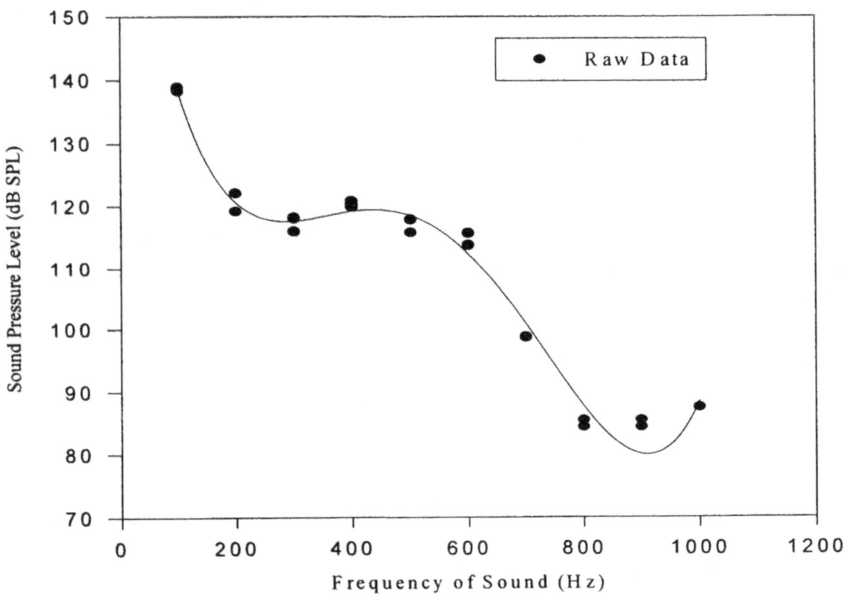

Figure 4. Calibration curve of test cell. Sound pressure level versus frequency of sound.

The dimensions of the hydrophone and test cell are such that the pressure levels detected by the hydrophone in the test cell can only be average values. Moreover, the behavior of Figure 4 is the combined effect of the behavior of the individual components of the sound generation system and the test cell, namely; the audio speaker, the piston, the size and stiffness of the diaphragms, and the size and volume of the test cell itself. From this perspective, the behavior of Figure 4 can be considered an *artifact* of the experimental setup, i.e., it has no connection with the mechanisms of the ear. It was necessary to obtain this data in order to determine the piezoelectric device sensitivities in later experiments.

Acoustic Impedance Matching Tests

The acoustic impedance of water is ~1.5 x 10^6 kg/(m^2-sec) and that of PZT 24 x 10^6 kg/(m^2-sec).[30] As a result of this large difference in the acoustic impedance of water and PZT, much of the sound pressure traveling in water and incident on the surface of a PZT device is reflected back into the water. Only the pressure that is transmitted into the ceramic results in the direct piezoelectric effect. Acoustic impedance mismatch, thus, causes a lowering in the transduction efficiency of a piezoelectric device. Moreover, in the case of the PZT devices, the ceramic was coated with Ag electrodes, which have an acoustic impedance ~ 36 x 10^6 kg/(m^2-sec). The greater acoustic impedance of Ag implies that an even smaller amount of pressure is transferred into the ceramic. The problem of acoustic impedance matching is usually overcome by placing one or more 'matching' layer(s) between the ceramic and the water.[31,32] Maximum impedance matching exists

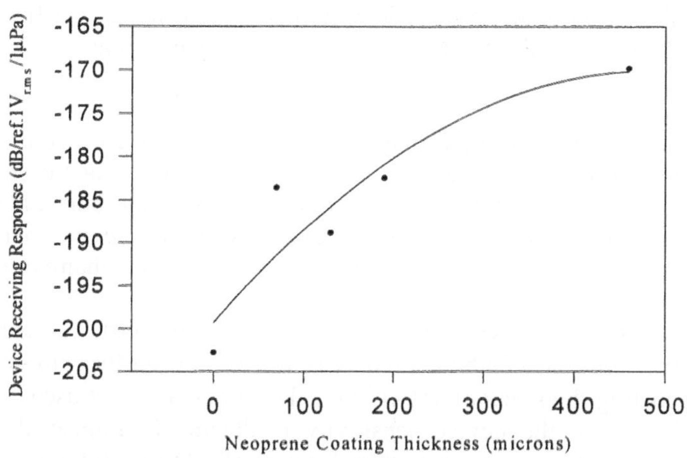

Figure 5. Plot showing the increase in device sensitivity of the PZT1 device as a result of increasing acoustic impedance matching.

when the matching layer thickness is nλ/4 (where: n = 1,3,5.... ; and, λ is the wavelength in the matching layer material).

Acoustic impedance matching tests were conducted on PZT chips of dimensions 5mm x 5mm x 0.260mm coated with neoprene rubber. Rubber has an acoustic impedance of ~1.0-2.5 x 10^6 kg/(m^2-sec). All measurements were conducted at a sound frequency of 600Hz. The neoprene layer thickness was gradually increased and measurements were taken at a distance of ~2mm $\pm$ 0.5mm from the front diaphragm. There was a scatter of $\pm$5mV in the measured values of the peak to peak voltage during these tests. Figure 5 shows the device receiving response (sensitivity) versus coating thickness behavior of a PZT1 device. From this plot, it is evident that the device sensitivity increases steadily with increased thickness of the Neoprene layer. This can be attributed to an improvement in impedance matching with increasing layer thickness. It must be mentioned that the layer thicknesses at which measurements were taken are far lower than the ¼λ layer thickness for sound of frequency 600Hz in Neoprene medium. It is significant that even at these thicknesses, conditions which can be referred to as 'far below resonance,' the improvement in device sensitivity with increasing layer thickness is dramatic.

Interestingly, the maximum sensitivity measured, ~ -170 dB (ref.1V_{rms}/1μPa), corresponds to a root mean square voltage of ~30mV across the electrodes of the device and a peak charge of ~8 x 10^{-11}C, four orders of magnitude greater than that predicted by a $-d_h$ based calculation for a PZT1 device of the same dimensions. Though the reasons behind such observations are not yet known, and all experimental station parameters and equipment and noise verified, they certainly strengthen the feasibility of a piezoelectric cochlear implant.

Voltage-Distance Tests

Voltage-distance tests were performed by placing the piezoelectric device in the test cell, near the center of the front diaphragm. Placement at this position allowed investigation of the nature of the acoustic waves in the bulk of the test station ('fast' waves),[8,9] away from the boundaries. Future experiments are planned in which the acoustic waves along the boundaries of the chamber ('slow' waves) will be investigated.[8,9,12]

The devices used for these tests were PZT piezoelectric ceramics of dimensions 5mm x 5mm x 0.260mm. Neoprene was coated on the wire-attached samples with a coating thickness of 450-490μm. This thickness was used because, as is seen in Figure 5, the device sensitivity is drastically improved at this thickness. Measurements were taken from a distance of ~2mm $\pm$ 0.5mm from the front diaphragm up to a distance of 30mm $\pm$ 1mm from the front diaphragm. At a distance of ~30mm from the front diaphragm, the device was ~2mm from the rear diaphragm. The noise level during the measurements was ~1mV.

The voltage-distance behavior of the PZT1 device at three frequencies is plotted in Figure 6. It is seen from this plot that the highest response is obtained at

600Hz. The response at frequencies above 600Hz was negligible. This can be explained by means of the calibration curve of Figure 4, in which it can be seen

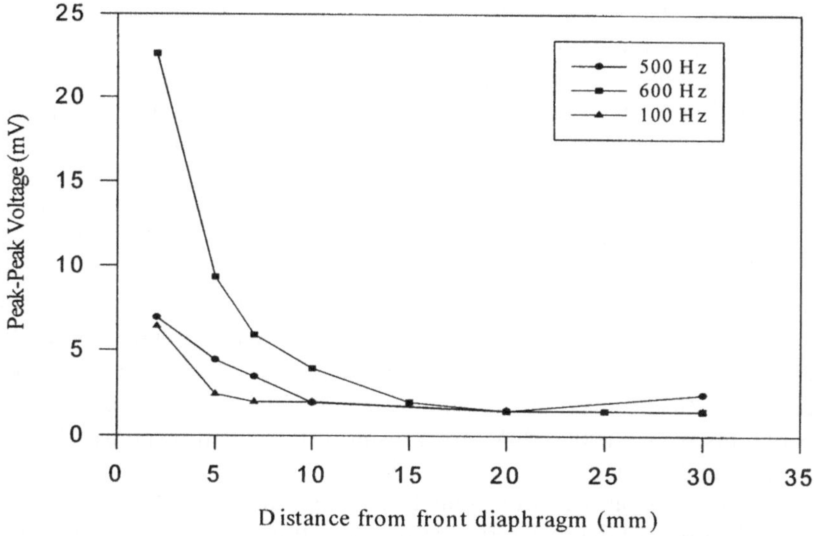

Figure 6. Plot showing the exponential decrease in sound pressures in the test cell.

that the sound pressure levels in the test cell drop sharply after 600Hz. From Figure 6 it is seen that the voltage detected by the device, and thus the sound pressure level in the test cell, decays exponentially with distance. In ideal free field sound conditions, the intensity of sound emanating from a spherical source varies as the inverse square of the distance (spherical dispersion).[38] The dimensions of the test cell are such that free field conditions are not expected to exist: hence the observed exponential decay. Another significant feature of the plots in Figure 5 is that, irrespective of the frequency of sound, the sound pressure level decays exponentially with distance. The difference in response of the piezoelectric device to frequencies below 600Hz, inspite of the fact that the sound pressure level at these frequencies is more or less constant (refer Figure 4), can be explained thus: The sound frequencies used for the test cell measurements imply wavelengths of several meters in the Neoprene. The wavelength of sound at 600Hz is 6 times smaller than the wavelength at 100Hz. Though still far thinner than quarter wavelength thickness, the 450-490μm thick Neoprene coating on the PZT device would be expected to provide better impedance matching for a 600Hz wave compared to a 100Hz wave. Hence the higher sensitivity at 600Hz. Other factors responsible for the observed sensitivity-frequency data of the PZT device include the inherent frequency response of the ceramic, the dimensions of the device, electrode type and thickness, and the presence of the Cu wires attached to the surface. Further experiments are planned in future to determine the effects of the above mentioned factors on the frequency sensitivity behavior of the device.

The results from the voltage-distance tests can be related to the events occurring in the cochlea. The vibrating stapes, lying against the oval window, produces a sound pressure wave in the scala vestibuli, which would be expected to suffer an exponential decay in intensity with increasing distance from the oval window.

Experiments were also conducted with PZT samples of dimensions 2mm x 1mm x 0.260mm. These piezoelectrics were also electroded with 25μm thick Ag electrodes and Cu wires were attached by the same procedure as was used for the larger samples. For these tests, devices with an ~100μm thick Neoprene coating were used. The voltage response, and the calculated charge densities on the electrodes (~0.036 $\mu C/m^2$), were much lower than that of the larger samples (~3.22 $\mu C/m^2$), with the maximum response being ~1mV. The noise levels for these experiments were ~100-200μV. As a result of this small response, detailed testing of these small devices were not carried out.

Theoretically speaking, if: a) the sound intensity (energy/unit area/unit time) in the testing chamber; b) the dielectric and piezoelectric constants of the ceramic; and, c) the type of electrode, remain unchanged, the charge density produced on the electrodes as a result of the direct piezoelectric effect should remain unchanged. The sound intensities used for tests with both the large and small samples were the same and the samples were all of the same composition. The charge density produced in the case of the smaller samples were, however, much lower than those produced by the larger samples. Though not yet proven, it is believed that this discrepancy arises as a result of the Cu wires, attached to both small and large samples in order to measure the voltage produced on the electrode surface. The wire size used was the same irrespective of the size of the piezoelectric. As a result, the joint between the wire and the electrode, which occupied only a small fraction of the electrode surface area in the case of the 5mm x 5mm samples, covered a larger area of the surface in the case of the smaller 2mm x 1mm samples. Consequently, the weight of the Cu wire and the Ag paste of the joint would be expected to play a greater role towards the physical clamping of the smaller piezoelectric as compared to that of the larger device. Hence the lower piezoelectric response in the case of the smaller device. This explanation is believed to be true as initial *in vivo* implantation of transducers of approximately this size in the cochlea of deafened guinea pigs resulted in positive auditory brainstem responses (ABR).[23]

CONCLUSIONS

- A mechanical analogue of the cochlea, an external test cell, was fabricated. This cell provided important data regarding cochlear acoustics and the feasibility of the use of piezoelectric devices as possible auditory nerve stimulators and as devices to investigate cochlear acoustics.
- Impedance matching plays an extremely vital role in determining piezoelectric device sensitivity and may prove to be critical for the fabrication of devices suitable to this application.
- The sound pressure level in the test cell was observed to decrease exponentially with increasing distance from the point of generation.
- This study, along with the initial work by Roseman, Willging, Wang, Buchanan, and Dong, is the first known effort attempting to implant piezoelectric devices in the cochlea of the profoundly deaf, with the purpose of exciting surviving auditory nerve fibers. Though theoretical calculations predict otherwise, results obtained from experiments in the test cell have shown encouraging results for feasibility of this device. Also, initial studies have proved that piezoelectric devices offer a novel and very useful means of investigating the acoustical phenomena in the mammalian cochlea.

ACKNOWLEDGEMENTS

The authors would like to thank Dr. R.C. Buchanan and Drs. Y.L. Wang (Shanghai Institute of Ceramics) and R.H. Dong (Huashan Hospital, Shanghai Medical College) for their suggestions and encouragement and initial research work at the University of Cincinnati. This research was sponsored by the University of Cincinnati Biomedical Research Fund.

REFERENCES

[1] G. von Bekesy, *Experiments in Hearing.* Wiley, New York, 1960.

[2] J.J. Zwislocki, "Five Decades of Research on Cochlear Mechanics," *J. Acoust. Soc. Am.,* 67 [2] 1679-1685 (1980).

[3] T.J. Glattke, "The Inner Ear: Anatomy and Physiology," in *Medical Audiology – Disorders of Hearing.* Edited by F.N. Martin. Prentice-Hall, New Jersey, 1981.

[4] J.O. Pickles, "The Physiology of the Cochlea," in *Cochlear Implants.* Edited by R.F. Gray. Croom-Helm, London, 1985.

[5] A.J. Hudspeth, "The Cellular Basis of Hearing: The Biophysics of Hair Cells," *Science*, 230 745-52 (1985).

[6] L.G. Johnsson, "Cochlear Anatomy and Histopathology," in *Cochlear Implants.* Edited by R.F. Gray. Croom-Helm, London, 1985.

[7] V. Nedzelnitsky, "Sound Pressures in the Basal Turn of the Cat Cochlea," *J. Acoust. Soc. Am.*, 68 [6] 1676-89 (1980).

[8] E.S. Olson, "Observing Middle and Inner Ear Mechanics with Novel Intracochlear Pressure Sensors," *J. Acoust. Soc. Am.*, 103 [6] 3445-63 (1998).

[9] A. Dancer, A. Franke, "Intracochlear Sound Pressure Measurements in Guinea Pigs," *Hearing Research*, 2 191-205 (1980).

[10] E. Fuhrman, W. Schneider, and M. Schultz, "Wave propagation in the Cochlea (Inner Ear): Effects of Reissner's Membrane and Non-Rectangular Cross Section," *Acta Mechanica*, 70 [1-4], 15-30 (1987).

[11] C. Cancelli, S. D`Angelo, and M. Masili, "Experimental results in a Physical Model of the Cochlea," *J. Fluid Mech.*, 153 361-388 (1985).

[12] L.C. Stenning, "Cochlear Mechanism: Theory Based on Slow Fluid Waves," *Acustica*, 44 135-147 (1980).

[13] J.B. Allen, "Cochlear Micromechanics – A Physical Model of Transduction," *J. Acoust. Soc. Am.*, 68 [6] 1660-1678, (1980).

[14] R.C. Black, G.M.Clark, and J.F. Patrick, "Current Distribution Measurements within the Human Cochlea," *IEEE Trans. Biomed. Engg.*, BME-28 [10] 721-24 (1981).

[15] *Cochlear Implants*, Edited by R.F. Gray. Croom-Helm, London, 1985.

[16] E. Feigenbaum, "Cochlear Implant Devices for the Profoundly Hearing Impaired," *IEEE Engineering in Medicine and Biology Magazine*, 6 [2] 10-21 (1987).

[17] W.F. House, "Cochlear Implants – Present and Future," *The Otolaryngologic Clinics of North America*, 19 [2] 217-18 (1986).

[18] R.P. Fravel, "Cochlear Implant Electronics Made Simple," *The Otolaryngologic Clinics of North America*, 19 [2] XI-XXII (1986).

[19] R.L. White, "System Design of a Cochlear Implant," *IEEE Engineering in Medicine and Biology Magazine*, 6 [2] 42-46 (1987).

[20] M. Soma, F.A. Spelman, and J.T. Rubinstein, "Fields Produced by the Cochlear Prosthesis: The Ear as a Multilayered Medium," *Procs. 6th Ann. Conf. IEEE Engg. in Med. and Bio. Soc.*, 401-405 (1984).

[21] C.N. Jolly, F.A. Spelman, and B.M. Clopton, "Quadrupolar Stimulation for Cochlear Prostheses: Modeling and Experimental Data," *IEEE Trans. Biomed. Engg.*, 43 [8] 857-65 (1996).

[22] K.J. Dormer, M.A. Phillips, "Auditory Prostheses: Implantable and Vibrotactile Devices," *IEEE Eng. in Med. and Biol. Mag.*, 6 [2] 36-41 (1987).

[23] N. Mukherjee, R.D. Roseman, and J.P.Willging, "The Piezoelectric Cochlear Implant: Concept, Feasibility, Challenges, and Issues," submitted to the *Journal of Biomedical Materials Research*.

[24]G.H. Haertling, "Piezoelectric and Electro-optic Ceramics", in *Ceramic Materials for Electronics*, 2nd ed. Edited by R.C. Buchanan. Marcel Dekker, New York, 1991.

[25]C.B. Sawyer, "The use of Rochelle salt Crystals for Electrical Reproducers and Microphones," reprinted from *IRE Proc.*, 19 2020-29 (1931). In *Acoustic Transducers.* Edited by I. D. Groves, Jr. Hutchinson Ross, Stroudsburg, 1981.

[26]M. Tamura, T. Yamaguchi, T. Oyaba, and T. Yoshimi, "Electroacoustic Transducers with Piezoelectric High Polymer Films," reprinted from *Audio Eng. Soc. J.*, 23 21-26 (1975). In *Acoustic Transducers.* Edited by I. D. Groves, Jr. Hutchinson Ross, Stroudsburg, 1981.

[27]R.E. Newnham, D.P. Skinner, and L.E. Cross, "Connectivity and Piezoelectric-Pyroelectric Composites," *Mat. Res. Bull.*, 23 525-36 (1978).

[28]K.A. Klicker, W.A. Schulze, J.V. Biggers, "Piezoelectric Composites with 3-1 Connectivity and a Foamed Polyurethane Matrix," *Communications of the American Ceramic Society*, C-208 (1982).

[29]A.J. Lovinger, "Ferroelectric Polymers," *Science*, 220 1115-21, (1983).

[30]H.R. Gallantree, "Review of Transducer Applications of Polyvinylidene Fluoride," reprinted from *IEE Procs.*, 130 219-24 (1983). In *Piezoelectricity.* Edited by C.Z. Rosen, B.V. Hiremath, and R.E. Newnham, American Institute of Physics, New York, 1992.

[31]G. Kossoff, "The Effects of Backing and Matching on the Performance of Piezoelectric Ceramic Transducers," *IEEE Trans. Sonics Ultrasonics*, SU-13 20-30 (1966).

[32]L.M. Brekhovskikh, *Waves in Layered Media.* Translated from Russian by D. Lieberman. Academic Press, New York, 1960.

[33]F.A. Spelman, B.M. Clopton, and L.G. Duckert, "Biophysical and Physiological Mechanisms for the Encoding of Speech through a Cochlear Prosthesis," *Procs. 6th Ann. Conf. IEEE Engg. in Med. and Bio. Soc.*, 406-10 (1984).

[34]W.G. Cady, *Piezoelectricity*, 1st edition. McGraw Hill, New York, 1946.

[35]B. Jaffe, W. Cook Jr., and H. Jaffe, *Piezoelectric Ceramics*, Academic Press, New York, 1971.

[36]*Piezoelectric Ceramics.* Product Brochure, EDO Corp., Acoustics Division, Salt Lake City, UT, USA.

[37]S.A. Shamma-Donoghue, G.A. May, N.E. Cotter, R.L. White, and F.B. Simmons, "Thin-Film Multielectrode Arrays for a Cochlear Prosthesis," *IEEE Trans. Elec. Dev.*, ED-29 [1] 136-44 (1982).

[38]V.M. Albers, *Underwater Acoustics Handbook*, Pennsylvania State University Press, 1960.

Characterization of plasma sprayed HA/ZrO_2 Composite Coatings

L. FU, K. A. KHOR, V. J. P. LIM
School of Mechanical and Production Engineering
Nanyang Technological University
Singapore 639798

ABSTRACT

In this study, yttria stabilized zirconia has been applied to reinforce hydroxyapatite coatings. HA/YSZ composite powders have been prepared by plasma spraying processing. Zirconia-reinforced hydroxyapatite coatings were characterized using X-ray diffraction (XRD), Fourier transform infrared spectroscopy (FTIR), scanning electron microscopy (SEM) equipped with an energy-dispersive X-ray analyzer (EDX). The addition of zirconia proved to be beneficial to reduce the other phases (CaO, TCP,TTCP) formation in the coatings. Meanwhile, a trace of $CaZrO_3$ formed in the coatings. A significant improvement in mechanical properties was achieved.

1. Introduction

Medical applications of ceramics have seen a rapid development in recent years. Hydroxyapatite(HA), $Ca_{10}(PO_4)_6(OH)_2$ in the form of calcium phosphate is a bio-ceramic material that has favorable osteoconductive and bioactive properties which promotes rapid bone formation and strong biological fixation to bony tissues[1]. Plasma sprayed HA coatings on metallic substrates have been developed for the use of medical and dental implants to improve the poor mechanical properties that the bulk hydroxyapatite materials possess [2]. The bone bonding capability of HA is also related to the surface porosity. A surface with macropores larger than 100μm is known to help bone to grow into the structure [3]. Thus by applying a porous coatings of HA on mental substrate, one can produce a biocompatible surface that can bond directly to bone. Other advantages of having the coating/substrate assembly include reduced metallic ion release in the physiological environment [4], and better mechanical stability of the assembly due to the tougher nature of metals. But the poor bond strength between the coatings and substrate has been the point of potential weakness in prothesis.

The long-term stability of a coating is more important when the influence of a physiological medium is considered. Therefore, to bridge the gap in HA coatings having low bond strength, bio-ceramic composite coatings are being developed. Zirconia (ZrO_2), having the attributes of high strength and stress-induced phase transformation toughening, has been used to strengthen the brittle materials [5-7]. In this work, yttria-stabilized zirconia has been used to reinforce the HA coatings. The microstructure characterization of the composite coatings has been studied. Efforts were made to know the influences of zirconia addition to the HA coatings.

2. Experimental procedure

2.1 Plasma spraying

HA/ZrO_2 mixed powders have been prepared by ceramic slurry method. A detailed description of this method was reported in earlier work [8,9]. This approach in preparing HA/ZrO_2 mixed powders was to utilize a ZrO_2 ceramic slurry (The particle size of zirconia is about 3 microns) to coat a layer of ZrO_2 particles on the HA powders (The average particle size of HA is about 35 microns). The mixed HA/ ZrO_2 aggregates contained 30wt% ZrO_2. Spherical HA/ZrO_2 particles were produced by plasma spraying into a tank of distilled water. The spheroidized powders were calcined at 800°C for 2 hours to transform the amorphous calcium phosphate into crystalline phase. Figure 1 is XRD pattern of the spheroidized powders. It reveals essentially pure crystalline HA and ZrO_2 in the spheroidized HA/ZrO_2 composite powders. Figure 2 shows the morphology and the cross-section microstructure of the spheroidized HA/ZrO_2 powders. It can be seen that some of zirconia is embedded in the HA to form HA/ZrO_2 mixtures and some is separate from HA.

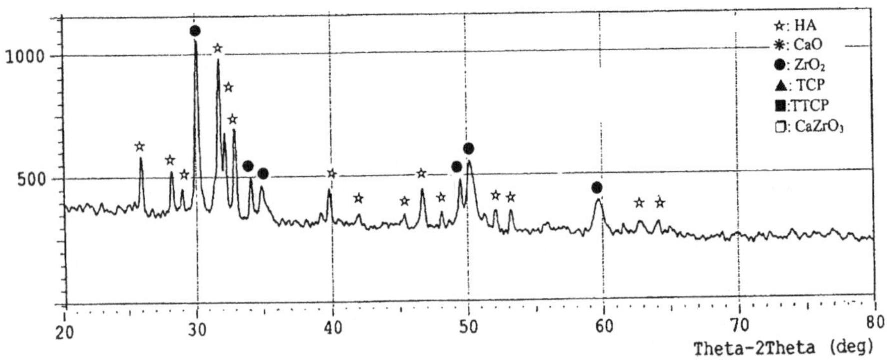

Figure 1. X-ray diffraction pattern of plasma spheroidized HA/ZrO_2 composite powders

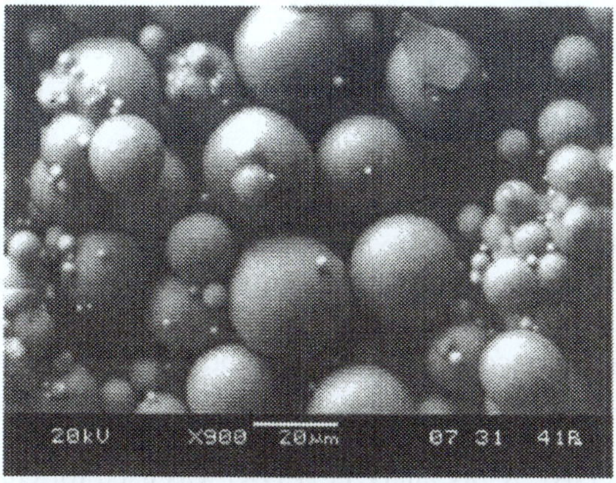

(a)

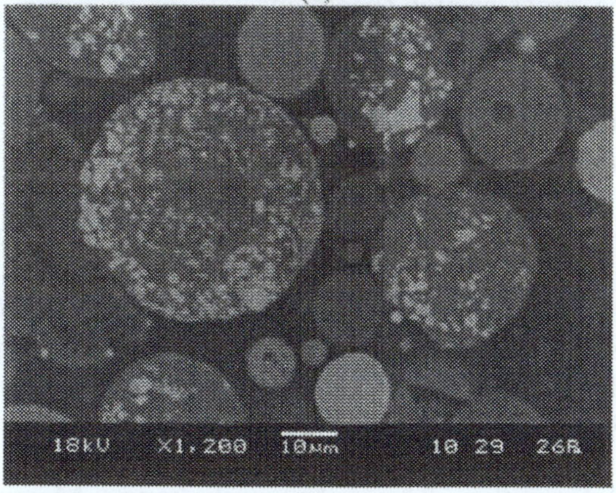

(b)

Figure 2. Scanning electron micrograph showing plasma spheroidized powders.
(a) morphology (b) cross-section

Table 1 Plasma spraying parameters

Net energy of plasma torch(kW)	10 – 15
Primary gas/Flow rate(m^3/h)	Ar/1.70
Secondary gas/Flow rate(m^3/h)	He/ 1.15
Powder feed rate(g/min)	10
Powder carrier gas/Flow rate(m^3/h)	Ar/0.25–0.85
Stand off distance (cm)	10
Substrate	Ti-6Al-4V

The substrates used for the coatings were Ti-6Al-4V alloy. They were sand blasted using silicon carbide grits and then ultrasonically cleaned. A 100kW net energy computerized control plasma system coupled with a robot unit (Praxair Surface Technologies, USA) was used to ensure control and repeatability of the plasma spraying process. The parameters used for plasma spraying are listed in Table 1

2.2 Microstructure characterization analysis

The phase analysis of the coatings was carried out using Philip MPD 1880 X-ray diffractometer with Ni-filtered Cu Kα radiation at 40kV and 30mA. The 2θ range from 20° to 80° was covered at a step size of 0.02° min^{-1}. Fourier transform infrared spectroscopy spectra were obtained using Perkin ALMER system 2000 FT-IR to observe the structure alteration which occurred during the plasma spray process. The Jeol scanning electron microscope equipped with an energy-dispersive X-ray analyzer (EDX) was used for characterization of the coating surface, cross-section specimens.

3. Results and discussions

3.1 Phase composition of HA/ZrO_2 coatings

Figure 3 is XRD pattern of the as-sprayed HA/ZrO_2 composite coating. It indicates that coating consists of crystalline HA, tetragonal zirconia, a little amount of calcium oxide (CaO), tricalcium phosphate (TCP), tetracalcium phosphate (TTCP) and a trace of calcium zirconium oxide ($CaZrO_3$). Compared to the XRD pattern of pure HA as-sprayed coatings (Figure 4) which obtained at the same plasma spraying parameters, it can be found that the amount of CaO, TCP, TTCP decreased greatly with the addition of zirconia. It reveals that the addition of zirconia can reduce the other phases (CaO, TCP, TTCP) formation during plasma spraying. Meanwhile, a new phase of $CaZrO_3$ formed in the coatings.

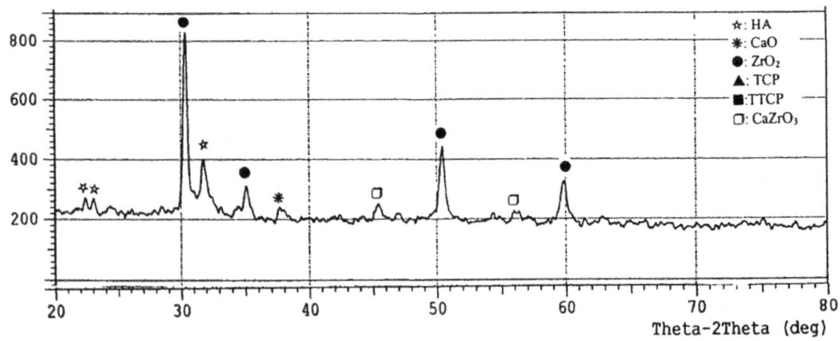

Figure 3 XRD pattern of the as-sprayed HA/ZrO_2 composite coating

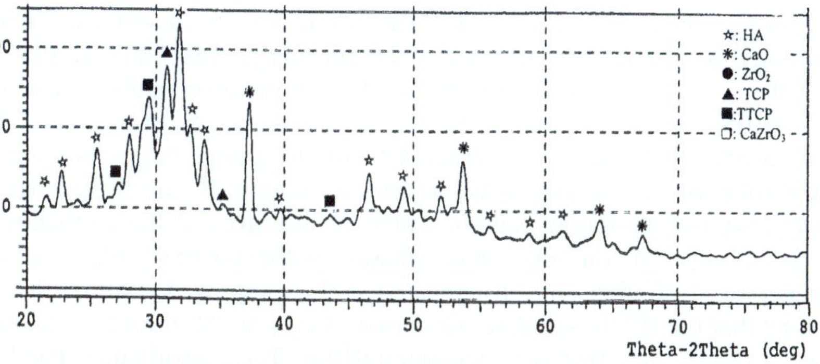

Figure 4 XRD pattern of pure HA as-sprayed coating

This result is different from the previous works on bulk materials [10-12] and plasma spraying of HA/ZrO_2 [13]. HIP post-sintering of HA ceramics with tetragonal ZrO_2 showed that the CaO in HA diffuses into ZrO_2 to cause tetragonal ZrO_2 to transform into cubic ZrO_2. The loss of CaO will then accelerate the decomposition of HA to beta-tricalcium phosphate above 800°C[10]. Similar to the result of Ioku et al., Tamari et al. [11]hot pressed bulk materials at 1300-1400°C and also found the transformation of tetragonal ZrO_2 into cubic ZrO_2 phase after sintering, but α-TCP was the decomposition product rather than β-TCP phase. Another study by Wu and Yeh [12]indicated that at sintering temperatures over 1150°C, HA will decompose into β-TCP and CaO , ZrO_2 will further react with CaO to produce a new $CaZrO_3$ phase. Chang et al.[13] studied the plasma spraying of zirconia reinforced HA composite coatings with the addition of 5 and 10wt% of ZrO_2 stabilized by Y_2O_3. The results showed that ZrO_2 reacted with CaO in HA to form $CaZrO_3$ and accelerates HA decomposition to α-TCP and TTCP during plasma spraying. In our study, the small amount of tetracalcium phosphate (TTCP), tricalcium phosphate (TCP), and CaO in the XRD pattern of as-sprayed coating with 30wt% zirconia additive suggested that the Ca components in HA dissolved in the zirconia to form solid solution when HA and zirconia were melted and mixed at high plasma temperature. This dissolution procedure limited HA further decomposition. Meanwhile, CaO in HA reacted with ZrO_2 to form a new phase of $CaZrO_3$. After heat treatment, the amorphous phase recrystallized, TTCP and TCP were transformed to crystalline HA (Figure 5). It means that the hydrolysis reactions between TTCP, TCP and water molecules lead to the formation of HA.

Not only is the X-ray diffraction analysis important, in addition, the infrared spectra must be reviewed critically, since they can bring out the features that cannot be observed by XRD. The Fourier transform infrared spectroscopy (FTIR) spectra of the HA starting powder, as-sprayed coating and heat treated coating were shown in Figure 6. The clear, sharp absorbance bands demonstrated by the IR spectra for the HA starting powder indicate that the HA powder was crystalline (Figure 6(a)). The absorbance bands represented from 938-1056cm^{-1} are characteristic for the presence of $(PO_4)^{-3}$ ions. The absorbance band at 3566cm^{-1} is characteristic of OH group. Analysis of the IR spectra for the as-sprayed HA/ ZrO_2 composite coating (Figure 6(b)) revealed a broad phosphate stretching region, which is indicative of the formation of some amorphous calcium phosphate phases in the coating [14]. The OH absorbance band of 3566 cm^{-1} disappeared in the as sprayed coating, thereby suggesting that the HA has undergone dehydroxylation. All the above features can be assigned to oxyhydroxyapatite(OHA). The absorbance band of 3458cm^{-1} is the characteristic of absorbed water (H_2O). After heat treatment, the vacancy of the missing OH^- group reoccupied in HA lattice (Figure 6 (c)). It indicated that the HA recrystalline occurred during heat treatment.

It is important to point out that XRD analysis does not reveal the dehydroxylation of HA. The XRD patterns of the main components of both HA powders and the as-sprayed HA/ZrO_2 coating are apatitic structure patterns. If the structural characterizations were only based on XRD analysis, one could conclude to a hydroxyapatite structure. Yet, the recorded IR spectra of the as-sprayed coating do not correspond to that of HA, but resemble that of OHA. The information contained in the characteristic spectral features of the OH^- (3566cm^{-1}) group lead to the identification of important structural characteristics that can not be made by XRD.

3.2 Microstructure characterizations

Figure 7 is a scanning electron micro-graph of plasma-sprayed coating surface showing splats, pores and unmelted particles. The better molten state has been achieved. Most of the particles became droplets in plasma flame and attached drop by drop to form the coating. Because of the high melting point of zirconia (~2680°C) and the short heating time (10^{-3} s) in high temperature plasma, it is difficult to melt all the zirconia.

Figure 8 shows the cross-section microstructure of HA/ZrO_2 composite coating measured by back-scatter electron (BSE). The distinguishable laminar gradient color from white to dark in the coating represents the mixture with different content of zirconia. It indicates that the solid solution actually formed during plasma spraying. The results measured by EDX are given in Figure 9. Referring to EDX analysis, the white region is the mixture of zirconia with a little CaO. The dark region is HA or calcium phosphates. The different grey regions represent the mixtures of HA or calcium phosphates with different content of zirconia. There is some porosity and some unmelted zirconia in the cross-section microstructure. The interface between the coating and the substrate looks very well.

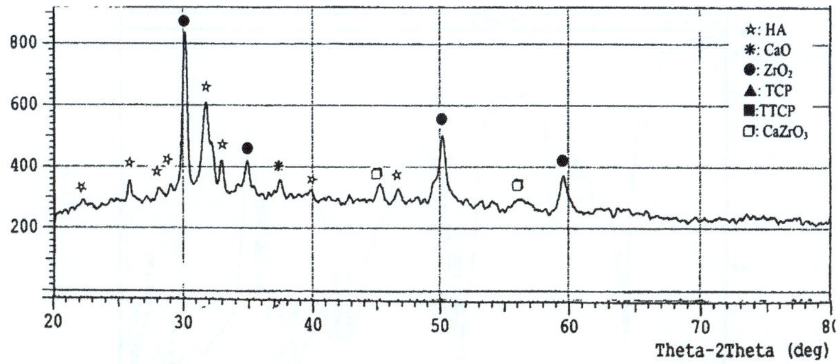

Figure 5. XRD pattern of the coatings heat treated at 800°C for 2 hours

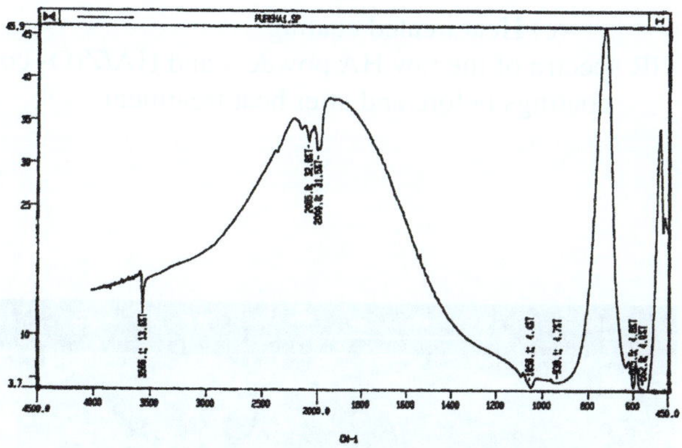

(a) FTIR spectrum of the raw HA powders

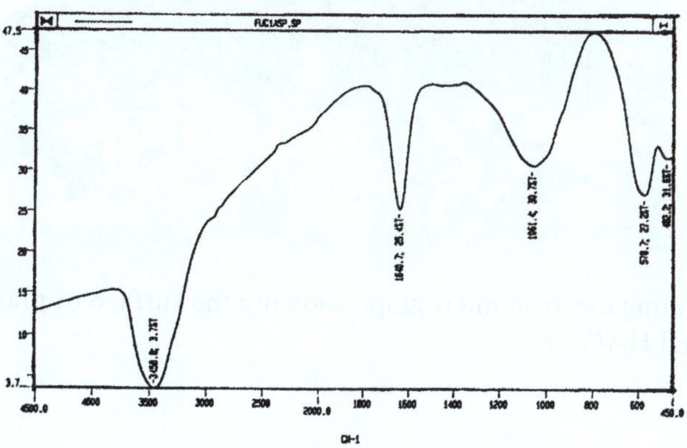

(b) As-sprayed HA/ZrO_2 coating

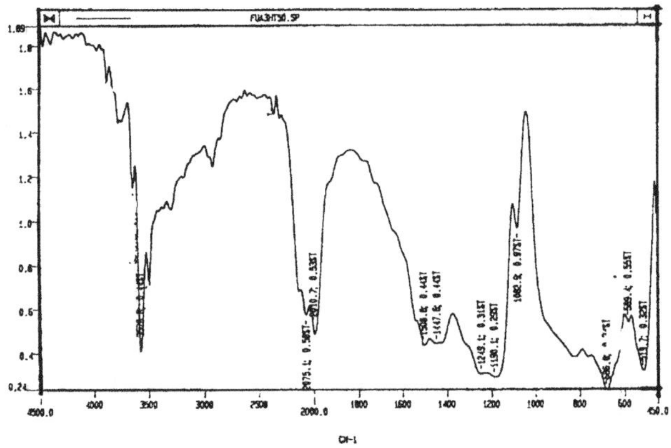

(c) Heat treated coating

Figure 6 FTIR spectra of the raw HA powders and HA/ZrO_2 composite coatings before and after heat treatment

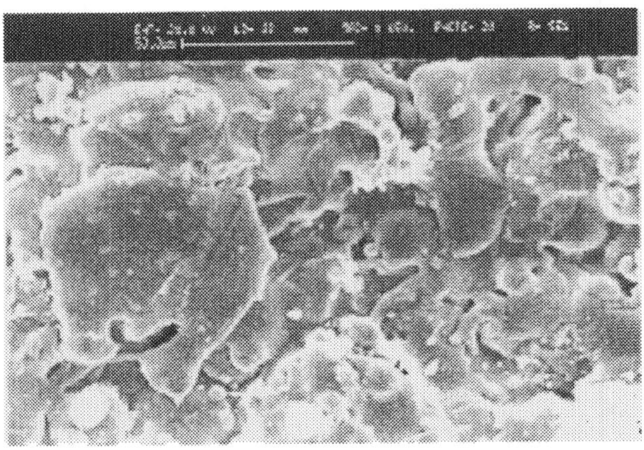

Figure 7 Scanning electron micrograph showing the surface of plasma-spray coated HA/YSZ

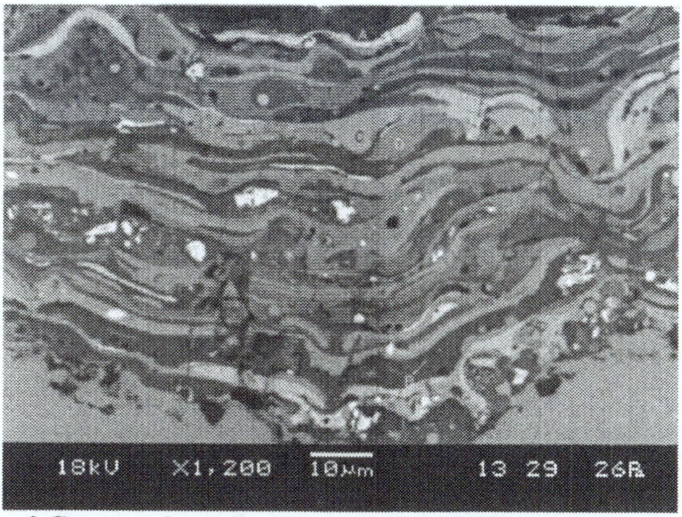

Figure 8 Cross-section microstructure of HA/YSZ composite coating

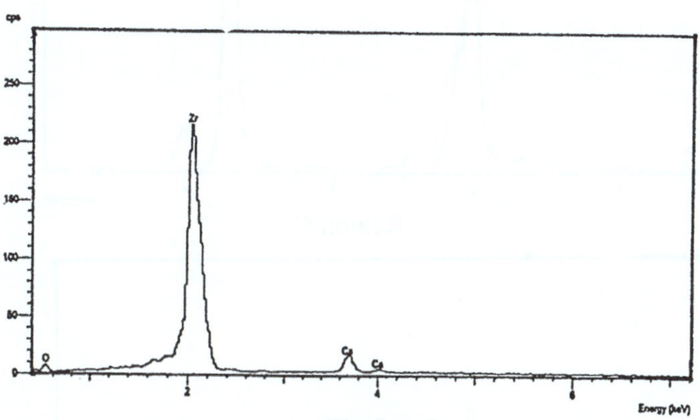

Region A

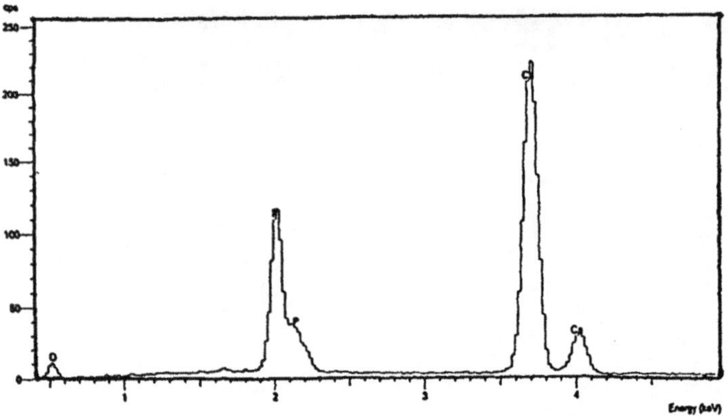

Region B

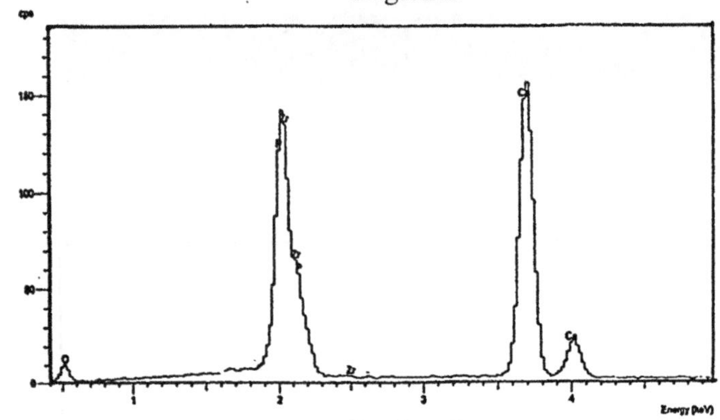

Region C

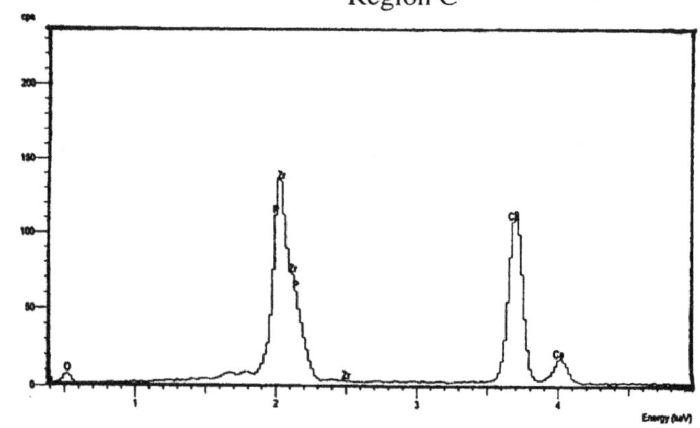

Region D

Figure 9 Element analysis of different regions measured by EDX

The comparison of the mechanical properties between HA coating and HA/YSZ composite coating has been shown in table 2. It shows that the bond strength and the Vicker hardness increase with the addition of zirconia. It also indicates that the positive effect of toughening by zirconia outweighed the negative effect such as increased porosity and unmelted zirconia particles. So the addition of zirconia reinforced the mechanical properties of HA coatings.

Table 2 Comparison of the mechanical properties of HA coatings and HA/ZrO2 composite coating

	HA Coatings	Composite coatings
Microhardness(MPa)	123.67	245.8
Bond Strength(MPa)	23.32	42.62

4 Conclusion

Characterization of plasma sprayed zirconia reinforced HA coating was performed by using XRD, FTIR, SEM equipped with EDX. The phases such as CaO, TCP and TTCP have been reduced greatly with the addition of zirconia. Meanwhile, a trace of $CaZrO_3$ formed during plasma spraying. HA/ZrO_2 composite coatings contain more unmelted small particles and increase the porosity in the coatings. The solid solution of HA with different content of zirconia formed. The tetragonal zirconia remains during plasma spraying. The mechanical properties of HA/YSZ composite coating have been improved. The positive effect of toughening outweighs the adverse effect of unmelted particles and increased porosity associated with the addition of zirconia.

References

1 H. Caulier, S. Vercaigne, I. Naert, J. P.C. M. Van der Waerden, J.G.C. Wolke, W. Kalk and J. A. Jansen, J. Biomed. Mat. Res., 34(1997), 147
2 M. Jarcho, Clin. Ortho. Rel. Res. 157(1981)259
3 E. Park, R. A. Condrate Sr., D. T. Hoelzer and G. S. Fischman, J. Mat. Sci. Mat. In Med., 9(1998)643
4 P. Ducheyne and K. Healy, J. Biomed. Mater. Res. 2(1988)1137
5 Q. L. Ge, T. C. Lei and Y. Zhou, Mater. Sci. Tech. 7(1991)490
6 Y. Murse, E. Kato and K. Daimon, J. Amer. Ceram. Soc. 69(1986)83
7 S. R. Witek and E. D. Butler, J. Mater. Sci. Lett. 4(1985)1412
8 C. S. Yip, K. A. Khor, N. L. Loh, P. Cheang, J. Mater. Proc. Tech., 65(1997)73
9 K. A. Khor, F. Y. C. Boey and T. Sano, J. Mater. Proc. Tech., 37(1993)431
10 K. Ioku, S. Somiya and M. Yoshimura, J. Jpn. Ceram. Soc. 99(1991)196

11 N. Tamari, M. Mouri and I. Kondo, J. Jpn. Ceram. Soc. 95(1987)806
12 J. M. Wu and T.S. Yeh, J. Mater. Sci, 23(1988)3771
13 E. Chang, W. J. Chang, B.C. Wang and C.Y. Yang, J. Mater. Sci. Mater. in Med., 8(1997)193
14 R.T. Bailey and C. Holt, Fourier Transform Infrared Spectroscopy and Characterization of Biological Calcium, CRC Press, Inc, Boca Raton, 1989, p93-120

OXIDE CERAMICS WITH CALCIUM PHOSPHATE COATINGS

J.Cihlar*, M.Jez, K.Castkova and M.Trunec
Technical University of Brno
Technicka 2, 61669 Brno
Czech Republic

ABSTRACT

Alumina, zirconia toughened alumina (ZTA), alumina toughened zirconia (ATZ) and zirconia ceramics were prepared by injection moulding. The surface of these ceramics was treated by applying layers of Ca-phosphates by the dip-coating method, or by infiltrating the surface of ceramics by the liquid Ca-phosphate precursor. Coatings of tricalcium phosphates were obtained that adhered well to the ceramic surfaces. Mechanical properties of the ceramics and the structure of coatings were studied by mechanical testing, XRD and SEM. Calcium phosphate coatings had little influence on the flexural strength and hardness of the ceramics but an increase in fracture toughness of coated ceramics could be observed.

INTRODUCTION

Ceramic components of joint implants made of aluminium oxide or zirconium dioxide have excellent mechanical properties but they lack bioactivity, which is in some cases (e.g. in the femoral component of the knee joint) very important. We believe that composite materials based on aluminium oxide and zirconium dioxide with Ca-phosphate (Ca-P)-based coatings could have not only good mechanical properties but also sufficient surface bioactivity. The method that lends itself to the preparation of Ca-phosphate coatings is the dip-coating method which, unlike the classical plasma coating, provides for the preparation of coatings of defined chemical and phase compositions. The infiltration of metallic matrix by the liquid phase is a procedure that has been used in the preparation of metalloceramic composite materials for several decades. Recently, the procedure has also been used in the preparation of ceramic composite materials with the aim of increasing their fracture toughness [1,2,3]. However, the infiltrations treated of in the present paper are not aimed at increasing the fracture toughness of oxide ceramic materials. The infiltration of oxide ceramics by Ca-phosphate precursors should increase the biocompatibility of the surface of bioinert ceramics or possibly ensure firm cohesion between the surface of bioinert ceramics activated by Ca-phosphates, and other, e.g. hydroxyapatite coatings. It remains to be seen, however, whether the treatment of the surface of oxide ceramics by applying Ca-phosphate coatings or by infiltration will or will not negatively affect the physical and mechanical properties of the ceramics that have been treated. The present work therefore focuses on the study of the effects of treating the surface of oxide ceramics by Ca-phosphate precursors on their mechanical properties, i.e.hardness, flexural strength and fracture toughness.

MATERIALS AND METHODS

Preparation of hydroxyapatite in water-alcohol sol of Ca-phosphate precursor

Isopropylester of phosphoric acid was prepared by the reaction of phosphorous pentoxide with anhydrous i-propanol [4]. The reaction product containing a mix of mono- and diisopropylester (molar ratio 1:1) then reacted with water solution of calcium acetate (Fluka) at a Ca/P molar ratio of 1.67. Added to the resulting water-alcohol sol of Ca-phosphate precursor were 10 wgt % of hydroxyapatite (Fluka). Under constant stirring and ultrasound action a stable suspension was formed in one hour.

Synthesis of solutions of EDTA-based Ca-phosphate precursor

The solution of precursor was prepared by the reaction of ethylendiamin-tetraacetate acid (EDTA) (Fluka) with $Ca(NO_3)_2$ (Lachema) and $(NH_4)_2HPO_4$ (Lachema) in water medium and in the presence of ammonia. The Ca/P molar ratio in the reaction mass was 1.67. The reaction solution was thickened under vacuum to a concentration of 10 wgt % of Ca-phosphate.

Preparation of oxide ceramics for the application of coatings and infiltrations

Used for the application of coatings and infiltrations were oxide ceramics based on Al_2O_3 (type RC-HP DBM, Reynolds Chemicals), ZrO_2 (type TZ-3YS, Tosoh) and composite materials containing 85 wgt % of Al_2O_3 and 15 wgt % of ZrO_2 (type ZTA85, Mandoval), and 80 wgt % of ZrO_2 and 20 wgt % of Al_2O_3 (type ATZ80, Mandoval). Test specimens were prepared by injection moulding of ceramic suspension and they were in the shape of a disk of 42 mm in diameter and 2.1 mm in thickness. The process and conditions of injection moulding are given in [5]. Ceramic specimens designed for the application of coatings were sintered for 2 h at a temperature of 1530°C (Al_2O_3, ZTA) or 1500°C (ZrO_2, ATZ). The specimens designed for infiltration were first annealed at a temperature of 1000°C and only after infiltration were they fired under conditions as given above.

Application of coatings by the dip coating method

The application of Ca-P coatings by means of HA suspension in a water-alcohol solution of Ca-phosphate was performed on a DIP MASTER MODEL 200 (Chemat Technology, USA). The coatings were applied at a speed of 20 mm/min. When 5 coatings had been applied, they were sintered at a temperature of 1300°C.

Infiltration of ceramics

Injection moulded specimens of ceramics (annealed at 1000°C) were dipped for 12 hours in a closed vessel holding the solution of EDTA-based Ca-phosphate precursor. The specimens were then dried by infrared heater and sintered.

Phase structure analysis

The qualitative phase structure analysis was performed with the aid of a D-500 (Siemens) diffractometer in central semifocus (Bragg-Brentan) arrangement, by CoK_α radiation using a direction-sensitive detector. The qualitative phase composition of specimens was established with the help of the PPF1-ICDD-JCPDS database [6]. The semiquantitative determination of the phase contents was based on modelling the diffraction spectra by the XQPA92 program [7].

Microstructure analysis of coatings

The structure of the surface and fracture areas of coatings was studied by means of scanning electron microscopy using a JXA (Jeol) machine.

Measurement of mechanical properties

Flexural strength of ceramic materials was established in accordance with the ISO Standards in the biaxial flexural strength test [8]. To test the mechanical properties a universal computer-controlled Zwick Z020 testing machine was used.
To establish the *hardness* of ceramic materials, a Wolpert Diaspor 2Rc hardness tester was used in the Vickers configuration. The loading force was 98 N (10kp). Prior to measuring, the specimen surface was finished by grinding off the coatings and polishing the surface.
To measure the *fracture toughness* the indentation fracture (IF) method was applied, which is part of the Japanese JIS R 1607 Standard [9]. The *lengths of cracks* c propagating from the corners of Vickers indentation were evaluated microscopically. The value of fracture toughness K_{IC} of the given material was estimated by means of an empirical relation given in [10].

RESULTS AND DISCUSSION

Ceramics with Ca-P coatings

The microstructure of Ca-phosphate coatings was similar and did not depend on the chemical composition of oxide ceramics to which the coatings had been applied. Fig.1 shows the coating applied to a ZrO_2 disk. The coating is formed by sintered grains of up to 5 μm in size. The size of irregularly scattered pores is up to 5 μm. The coating thickness (around 5 μm) and its cohesion with the ceramic substrate are clear from Fig.2. Compared with hydroxyapatite coatings applied by plasma spraying the coatings prepared by the dip-coating method were more uniform (cf. Fig.3). RTG analysis has shown (see Fig.4) that the coatings contained either a single phase, β-tricalciumphosphate (coatings applied to ZTA

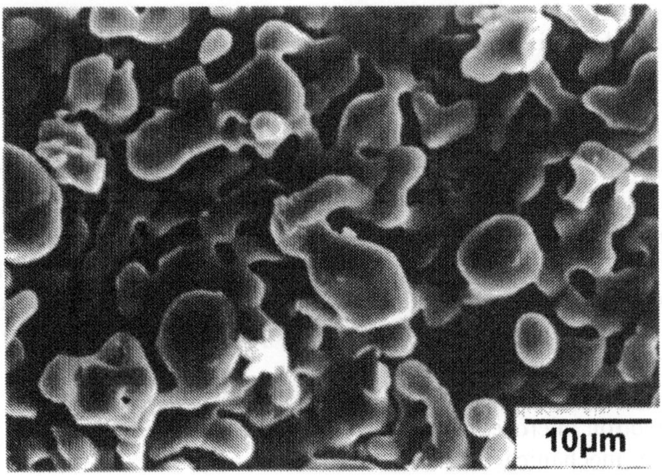

Fig. 1 Ca-phosphate coating on the surface of zirconia ceramics

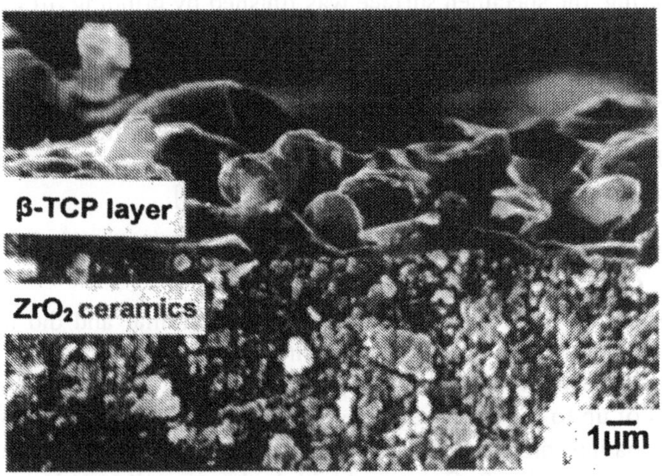

Fig. 2 Structure of the fracture surface of zirconia ceramics with applied Ca-phosphate coating

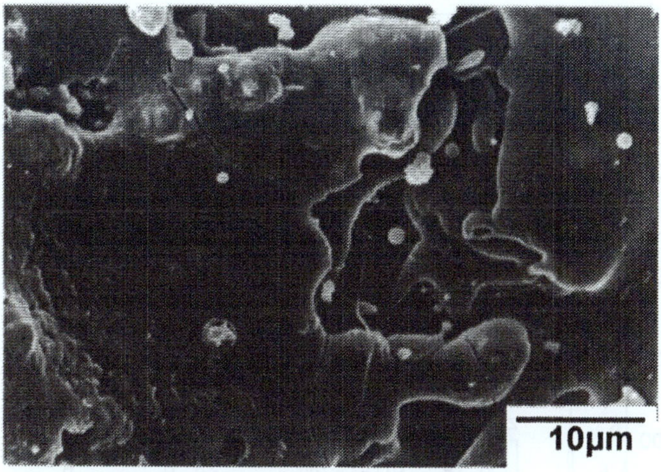

Fig. 3 Ca-phosphate coating applied to the surface of zirconia ceramics by plasma coating

and ATZ), or two phases, β-tricalciumphosphate and α-tricalciumphosphate (coatings applied to Al_2O_3 and ZrO_2). None of the coatings contained hydroxyapatite. According to our results [11] the pure hydroxyapatite ceramics decomposed thermally at the temperature higher than 1300°C. We therefore assume that the hydroxyapatite reacted with i-propylphosphate to form tricalciumphosphate. The adhesion of coatings to ceramic substrates (or the strength of the coating/ceramics interface) was not established but judging from the behaviour of coatings in hardness determination the cohesion between coatings and ceramics was good. When deforming the coatings by the Vickers indentor it never occurred that the coatings flaked off the ceramic substrate (see Fig.5). The *hardness* values of Al_2O_3, ZTA, ATZ and ZrO_2, given in Table 1, were not influenced by the Ca-P coating to any considerable degree. The highest hardness values of reference specimens, i.e. 16802 MPa, were obtained for Al_2O_3 and ZTA materials. Comparing these values with the values established for specimens with Ca-P coating there is a drop in hardness to 16174 MPa in Al_2O_3-based materials when compared with the reference specimen. In the case of ZTA no drop in hardness (16802 MPa) was established for the specimen with Ca-P coating in comparison with the reference specimen. ATZ exhibited the same hardness value, 13506 MPa, for both types of treatment. In the case of ZrO_2, the coating resulted in increased hardness. For specimens with Ca-P coating a value of 13052 MPa was established, and 11631 MPa for the reference specimens. The deviations measured for Al_2O_3 and ZrO_2 were small and they could be due to the

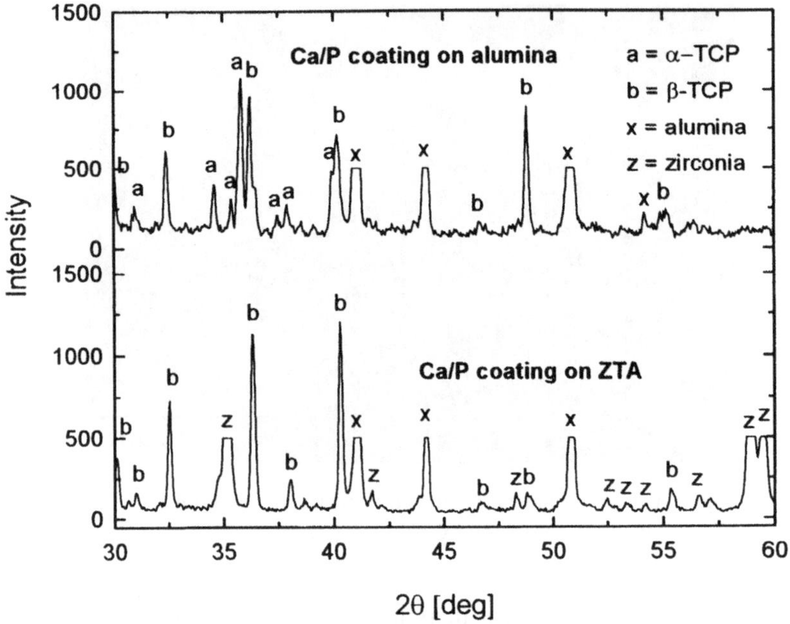

Fig. 4 XRD spectra of Ca-phosphate coatings

interactions of Ca^{2+} with Al_2O_3 and ZrO_2. However, the products of interaction, i.e. calcium aluminate and a higher content of t-ZrO_2 or c-ZrO_2, could not be evidenced by the phase analysis.

Biaxial flexural strength is given in Table 1. The effect of Ca-phosphate coatings on the strength (similar to the hardness) of oxide materials was small.

Table 1 Mechanical properties of ceramic materials with or without Ca-phosphate coatings

Ceramics	Flexural Strength [MPa]		Hardness [MPa]		Fracture toughness $[MPa \cdot m^{1/2}]$	
	without coating	with coating	without coating	with coating	without coating	with coating
Alumina	321.7	314.8	16802	16174	4.3	5.5
ZTA	431.0	408.5	16802	16802	5.0	5.9
ATZ	534.0	558.8	13506	13506	11.5	11.0
Zirconia	566.1	497.6	11631	13052	10.6	11.5

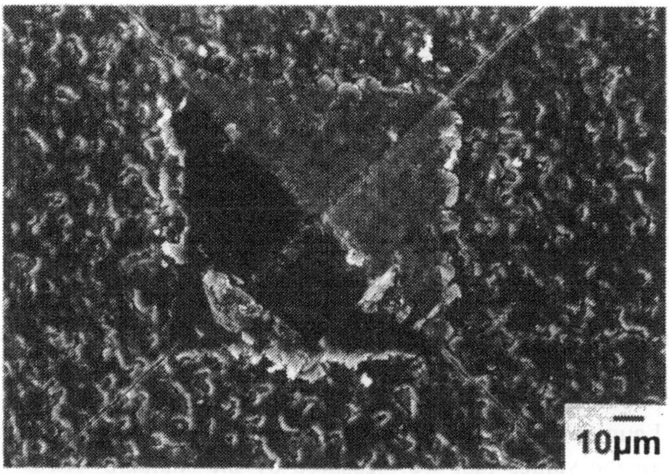

Fig. 5 Detail of indentation by Vickers indentor into a Ca-phosphate coating applied to ZTA ceramics

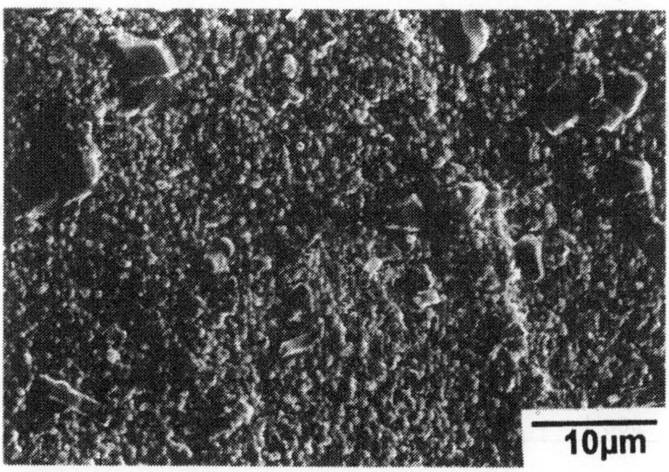

Fig. 6 Structure of the surface of infiltrated ATZ ceramics

In the case of Al_2O_3 the average strength value for the reference specimens was 321.7 MPa, for the coated specimens it was 314.8 MPa. In the case of ZTA, too, the strength of the reference specimen was higher (431.0 MPa). The applied Ca-P coating resulted in a strength reduction to 408.5 MPa. With ATZ the higher strength value was found for the coated specimens (558.8 MPa). The strength of reference material was a little lower (534.0 MPa). With ZrO_2 the highest strength was obtained for the reference material (566.1 MPa). The coated material had a lower strength (497.6 MPa). The markedly lower strength value of the coated ZrO_2 was probably due to the larger scattering of strength values.

For the measurement of *fracture toughness* the „Indentation Fracture" method was chosen because of its simplicity and the possibility of carrying out a great number of measurements. From a number of relations for the calculation of fracture toughness as published in the literature the most suitable proved to be the relation published by Laugier [10]. The values K_{IC} calculated by this relation were in good agreement with the values that we measured by the standard SEPB method on specimens with macrocracks. It is evident from the values of K_{IC} given in Table 1 that the coating had no marked effect on the fracture toughness of ceramic substrates.

Infiltrated ceramics

After the infiltration of porous ceramic materials based on Al_2O_3, ZTA, ATZ and ZrO_2 by EDTA-based liquid Ca-phosphate precursor a coating appeared on their surface whose typical structure can be seen in Fig.6). On the surface of infiltrated ceramics the presence of one or two phases - β-tricalciumphosphate and α-tricalciumphosphate – was established.

Table 2 Mechanical properties of ceramic materials infiltrated or uninfiltrated by Ca-phosphate precursors

Ceramics	Flexural Strength [MPa]		Hardness [MPa]		Fracture toughness [$MPa \cdot m^{1/2}$]	
	without infiltration	with infiltration	without infiltration	with infiltration	without infiltration	with infiltration
Alumina	321.7	320.1	16802	12210	4.3	6.9
ZTA	431.0	350.1	16802	15019	5.0	5.4
ATZ	534.0	495.3	13506	13506	11.5	23.2
Zirconia	566.1	553.3	11631	13052	10.6	14.6

The values of *biaxial flexural strength* of Al_2O_3, ZTA, ATZ and ZrO_2 are given in Table 2. The average strength value of Al_2O_3 reference specimens was 321.7 MPa, that of infiltrated specimens was 320.1 MPa. The average strength of non-infiltrated ZTA specimens was 431.0 MPa, after infiltration it dropped to 350.1

MPa. In the case of ATZ the higher strength was established for the reference material (534 MPa) in contrast to the infiltrated specimen, whose average strength was 495.3 MPa. With the ZrO_2 material the higher average strength was obtained for the reference specimen (566.1 MPa). Infiltration was of little effect on the strength, which dropped to 553.3 MPa. The infiltration of ceramics thus resulted in a slight reduction of strength. The reasons for the larger strength reduction in the case of ZTA (by about 20%) are probably mechanical (a greater amount of defects in ZTA prior to infiltration) and not chemical since infiltration practically did not affect the strength of single-component ceramics (Al_2O_3 and ZrO_2).
The *hardness* of Al_2O_3, ZrO_2, ZTA and ATZ materials is given in Table 2. The highest hardness of reference specimens, 16802 MPa, was measured for Al_2O_3 and ZTA. A comparison of these values with hardness values of materials subsequent to infiltration reveals for Al_2O_3 a drop to 12210 MPa. For ZTA the hardness of infiltrated material was found to drop from 16802 to 15019 MPa. This can be put down to the appearance of Ca-Al phases on the surface of Al_2O_3-based ceramics, whose hardness is lower than the hardness of pure α-Al_2O_3. The same hardness, 13506 MPa, was exhibited by ATZ for both types of treatment. The hardness of infiltrated ZrO_2 specimens increased to 13052 MPa, compared with the 11631 MPa established for the reference specimen.
The *fracture toughness* is given in Table 2 and in Fig.6. Evident from the K_{IC} values is the little effect of infiltration on the ZTA material (5.0 $MPa.m^{1/2}$ vs 5.4 $MPa m^{1/2}$). There was a slight increase for Al_2O_3 (4.3 $MPa.m^{1/2}$ vs 6.9 $MPa m^{1/2}$) and for ZrO_2 (10.6 $MPa m^{1/2}$ vs 14.6 $MPa m^{1/2}$). A marked increase in the fracture toughness appeared in infiltrated ATZ, where its increase was almost twofold (11.5 $MPa m^{1/2}$ vs 23.2 $MPa m^{1/2}$). The increase in fracture toughness observed in all types of infiltrated ceramics cannot be explained without a further study of infiltrated ceramics. On the basis of the results obtained we can assume a certain increase in fracture toughness in consequence of the „closing up" of surface defects or pores, or „healing" of the defects on grain boundaries. In the case of ATZ, however, these effects cannot explain the twofold increase in fracture toughness as compared with non-infiltrated material. We can only speculate on the cause of the above „toughening" - perhaps it is a combination of the optimum composite structure of ATZ, the hardening of grain boundaries during infiltration and the phase transformation of ZrO_2, which had the observed effect.

CONCLUSION

The study of oxide ceramic materials (Al_2O_3, ZTA, ATZ and ZrO_2) with coatings of Ca-phosphates has shown that Ca-P coatings were of no significant effect on hardness, flexural strength and fracture toughness. The infiltration of ceramic oxide materials by the EDTA-based liquid precursor of Ca-phosphate did not impair significantly their mechanical properties, i.e. hardness and strength. By contrast, fracture toughness increased in all cases (in the case of ATZ significantly). For a comprehensive description of the problems under study it will be necessary to complement the study by establishing the flexural strength of the interface between ceramic materials and Ca-P coatings, and by establishing the bioactivity of Ca-P coatings and infiltrated surfaces.

ACKNOWLEDGEMENTS

The authors thank D. Janova and Z. Vojtkulakova for SEM observations, and A. Buchal for XRD analysis. The research was supported by the Czech Ministry of Education, Grant No. VS96121.

REFERENCES

[1]J. Asaumi, H. Zoshida and N. Miyata, "Surface Modification of Mullite by Partial Infiltration of Zirconia," *J. Am. Ceram. Soc. of Japan., International Edition*, 98 52-9 (1990)

[2]D. Galusek and J. Majling, "Zirconia Based Organic Precursor Infiltration as a Method for Preparation of ZTA Ceramics, Pt.2. Sintering and Materials Behaviour," *Ceramics-Silikaty*, 40 23-4 (1996)

[3]J.G. Duh and J.U. Wan, "Liquid Infiltration in ZrO Sub 2 Ceramics," *J. Mater. Sci*, 12 473-5 (1993).

[4]J. Cihlar and K. Castkova, "Synthesis of Calcium Phosphates from Alkyl Phosphates by Sol-Gel Method," *Ceramics-Silikaty*, 42 [4] 164-70 (1998).

[5]M. Trunec and J. Cihlář, "Thermal Debinding of Injection Moulded Ceramics," *J. Eur. Ceram. Soc.*, 17 203-9 (1997).

[6]R. Jenkins et al (eds), in *Powder Diffraction File, Inorganic Phases,* JCPDS International Centre for Diffraction Data, Swarthomore 1987.

[7]L. Smrcok and J. Weiss, *J. Appl. Cryst.*, 26 140-1 (1993).

[8]"Implants for Surgery-Ceramics Materials Based on High Purity Alumina," ISO Standard No. 6474 (1991).

[9]"Testing Methods for Fracture Toughness of High Performance Ceramics," JIS R Standard No. 1607 (1990).

[10]M.T. Laugier, "The Elastic/Plastic Indentation of Ceramics," *J. Mater. Sci., Letters*, 4 1539-41 (195).

[11]J. Cihlář, A. Buchal and M. Trunec, "Kinetics of thermal decomposition of hydroxyapatite bioceramics", *J. Mater. Sci.,* in print.

PROCESSING, BIOCOMPATIBILITY AND BIOMECHANICAL TESTING OF POROUS ALUMINA CERAMICS

Susmita Bose[1], Jens Darsell[1], Lihua Yang[2], Dipak K Sarkar[2] and Amit Bandyopadhyay[1]
[1]School of Mechanical and Materials Engineering
[2]College of Veterinary Medicine
Washington State University
Pullman, WA 99164-2920

ABSTRACT

Ceramic materials that are used for the reconstruction or replacement of the damaged parts of the body are called Bioceramics. Bioceramic materials have been a great deal of interest for numerous applications to scientists, physicians as well as engineers for last four decades. In this present work, preparation, biocompatibility and mechanical testing of porous alumina and hydroxyapatite (HAp) coated alumina ceramics are also discussed. The biological responses of rat pituitary tumor cells (PR1) on these materials were assessed *in vitro*. All the materials provided favorable sites for cell attachments in a physiological solution at 37^0C which reveals that the materials may promote good bonding while used as bone implants.

INTRODUCTION

During past four decades, the use of ceramics has revolutionized the quality of human life. Many specialty ceramics and glasses have been developed for the use of the health care industry, e.g., eyeglasses, diagnostic instruments, thermometers, tissue culture flasks, carriers for enzymes and antibodies, and ceramics in dentistry as restorative material.[1-4] These novel ceramic materials that are used for the repair and reconstruction of diseased or damaged part of the musculo-skeletal system are called bioceramic materials. Due to their low density, chemical inertness, and compositional similarities with human tissues, bioceramic materials are preferred as bone graft over metals and composites. The potential of any bioceramic material to be used as an implant depends upon their biocompatibility with the physiological environment. Different ceramics have been tested for their use inside human body, however, only a few have achieved successful human clinical applications.

In general, bioceramic materials are classified in three broad categories based on their applications. They are (i) bioinert (alumina, zirconia), (ii) bioresorbable (tricalcium phosphate) and (iii) bioactive (hydroxyapatite, bioactive glasses, glass-ceramics). A bioinert material is nontoxic but biologically inactive, where as a bioactive material is the one that elicits a specific biological response at the interface of the biological part and the material, which results in the formation of a bond between the tissues and the material. The terms biodegradable, bioresorbable and bioabsorbable are often used interchangeably and indiscriminantly. A biodegradable substance can break down *in vivo*, but for a bioabsorbable material, the break down products are metabolized locally and systemically.[5,6]

Various bone substitutes that are currently being used include: (1) autograft (tissue from the another location from the body of the same individual), (2) allograft (tissue from different individuals of the same species), (3) genograft (tissue implnated from a different species) and (4) bone graft (artificial bone). Though autograft is probably the most suitable, it requires at least two operations and may result in patient morbidity (hemorrage, infection and pain). In both allograft and genograft, rejection by the patient's body and diseases transmitted by the foreign bone are of serious concern. Because of these reasons, applications of bone graft are becoming more and more used.

Bioceramic materials have been used for the replacements of hips, knees, teeth, tendons and ligaments, repair for periodontal disease, maxillofacial reconstruction, augmentation and stabilization of the jaw bone, spinal fusion and as a bone filler. Microporous implants have found a great deal of applications towards bone replacement studies. Porous bone implants with pore size in between 100-600 μm are found to be osteoconductive.[2] Advantages of using a porous implant is to increase the interfacial area between the implant and the tissue which results in less movement of the device in the tissue as well as provide blood supply to the connective in-grown tissue.

Various processing techniques have been utilized to fabricate porous ceramic scaffolds to enhance tissue regeneration and bone repair. The replamineform process was utilized to fabricate inert, bioactive, metallic and polymeric implants to duplicate the macroporous microstructures of corals that have interconnected pores.[7-9] In this approach, first natural corals are machined to the desired shapes. The machined coral is fired to drive off the carbon dioxide from the limestone leaving behind a calcia structure to be used as an investment material to form the porous structure. The desired material is then cast into the pores and the calcia mold is removed from the structure by dissolving it in dilute hydrochloric acid. Though the replamine process allow the fabrication of porous ceramic implants with pore size varying from 140 to 1000 μm, there is almost no control over the pore sizes, their distribution and their interconnectivity. The lack of flexibility in design and fabrication of controlled porosity bioceramic implants restrict the use of this process as a commercial process for mass production.

Porous alumina ceramics have also been fabricated using pore formers or foaming agents that evolve gases during sintering at elevated temperatures.[10-11] Porous Hydroxyapatite (HAp) ceramic blocks were also fabricated using a HAp slurry mixed with foaming agent followed by sintering at elevated temperature.[12] Unfortunately, all of these processes form structures with randomly arranged pores with a wide variety of sizes and have limited flexibility to control the pore architecture.

The present work will describe the processing and physical characteristics of controlled porosity alumina ceramics processed via rapid prototyping technique and their *in vitro* response towards PR1 rat pituitary tumor cells.

PROCESSING AND CHARACTERIZATION OF POROUS STRUCTURES

Processing of porous 3D honeycomb implants: 3D-honeycomb alumina ceramic preforms were fabricated using indirect fused deposition modeling process (FDM). FDM is one of the commercially available solid freeform fabrication (SFF) or rapid prototyping (RP) techniques commercialized by Stratasys® Inc. (Eden Prairie, MN) where thermoplastic polymeric materials are used to build three dimensional objects from their computer aided design (CAD) description. Solid freeform fabrication technologies emerged in the late 1980's as revolutionary manufacturing processes with the inherent capability to fabricate objects in virtually any shape without the need for molds, dies, or tooling. This is accomplished using various forms of material addition rather than material subtraction, a method common to nearly all conventional manufacturing processes (*e.g.* milling). The capabilities of SFF to rapidly fabricate small quantities of functional objects were quickly realized by high volume of manufacturers as an effective mechanism to streamline the time and cost of product development. As SFF has evolved to provide greater fabrication speed, improved accuracy, and access to engineering materials, it has become attractive to low volume manufacturers who benefit from direct fabrication in production materials.

The utilization of SFF processes to fabricate models derived from medical imaging data sources has received some attention in recent years. SFF was recognized by the surgical community as a potentially invaluable surgical tool to provide specific patient solutions. As such, SFF fabricated patient specific anatomical models have emerged as worthwhile tools for surgical planning as well as mechanisms of information dissemination to patients. In a classical application, James, *et al.*,[13] used SLA models to plan the surgical correction of a facial defect. Others have utilized the tooling capabilities of SFF to provide solutions to specific patient defects. Holle *et al.*,[14] discuss the use of an SLA model to plan surgical shaping and attachment of autograft implants. Erickson, *et al.*,[15] cast custom titanium orbital implants using wax patterns produced from SLA masters fabricated using medical imaging data.

However, SFF technology can be used to fabricate custom implantable scaffolds, which has tremendous potential to revolutionize treatment of skeletal defects. SFF, coupled with historically efficacious biomaterials, such as alumina and calcium phosphate based ceramics, potentially provides an optimal musculoskeletal reconstruction modality; one that can be tailored specifically to the indication. In addition, the virtually unlimited fabrication capabilities of SFF technology open vast opportunities for custom designed implant capabilities.

In this research, FDM, one of the SFF processes have been utilized to produce net shape controlled porosity alumina ceramic scaffolds. During FDM process, a thermoplastic polymer filament passes through a heated liquifier. The liquifier movement is computer controlled along the X and Y directions, based on the build strategy of the part to be manufactured. The liquifier extrudes a continuous bead, or road, of material through a nozzle and deposits it on a fixtureless platform. When deposition of the first layer is completed, the fixtureless platform indexes down, and the second layer is built on top of the first layer. This process continues until the fabrication of the part is completed. The temperatures of the liquifier and surrounding environment, as well as filament feed rate and nozzle diameter, are some of the important variables that determine the quality of the final part.[16] **Figure 1** shows the schematic of the FDM process. Porous ceramic implants using alumina (bio-inert) ceramic powders were fabricated using indirect FDM process. In the indirect route, the negative of the desired structure or mold was first fabricated via FDM. The positive was then cast using a ceramic slurry via lost mold technique.

Processing of porous 3D honeycomb alumina ceramic structures via indirect FDM consists of three stages of development and optimization work. They are:

(1) mold design, (2) development of ceramic slurry composition and (3) binder burn out and sintering cycle development for green ceramic structures.

Molds were designed and fabricated by FDM 1650 using commercially available ICW-06 filament material. Cylindrical molds were designed and fabricated with a (45/-45) raster filling and varying the raster gap from 0.625 to 1.2 mm (X and Y gap in Figure 2a). Top 6.25 mm of the mold had only perimeter but no raster filling, which is also called lip, to hold excess ceramic slurry during infiltration. Bottom four layers of the mold had no raster gap to avoid leaking of slurry during infiltration. Road width was varied from 0.375 to 0.625 mm. Combination of raster gaps and road widths control the volume fraction of ceramics and its pore sizes in the preform.

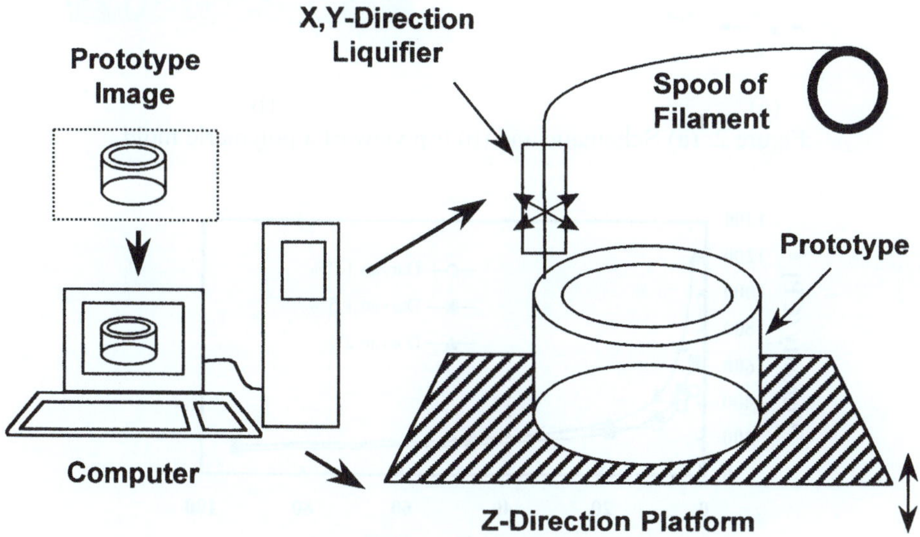

Figure 1: Schematic of fused deposition process

Development of ceramic slurry work started with various commercially available alumina powders. Finally most of the work had been performed with 6D, 10D and 30D alumina powders doped with 500 ppm of MgO (Baikowski International Corporation, NC). All the powders had submicron size particles, but specific surface areas were different for different powders. High surface area powder increases the slurry viscosity compared to low surface area powder at similar solids loading. Brookfield Viscometer was used to determine the optimum wt% of dispersant needed for the preparation of water based ceramic slurry by measuring the viscosity at different shear rates for each solution. 1-Butanol

(Fisher Scientific) was used as an antifoaming agent for these ceramic slurries. Darvan 821 (R.T. Vanderbilt & Co., Norwalk, CT) was found to be the best dispersant. For the 10D alumina powder, 1.5 wt% darvan was found to be optimum. Figure 3 shows the variation of slurry viscosity as a function of dispersant amount with respect to shear rate for 10D powders.

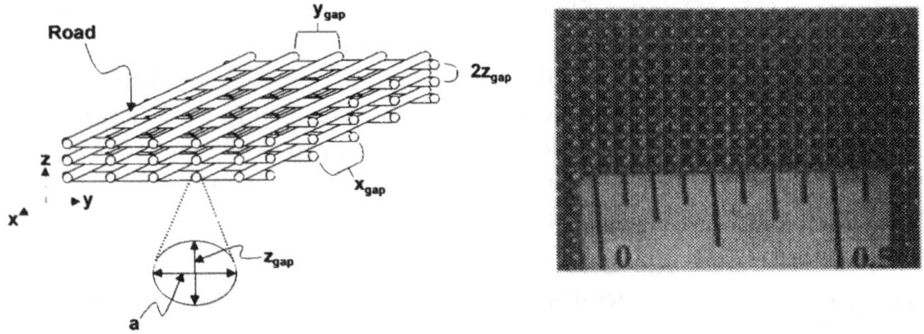

(a) (b)

Figure 2: (a) Schematic and (b) top view of a polymeric mold

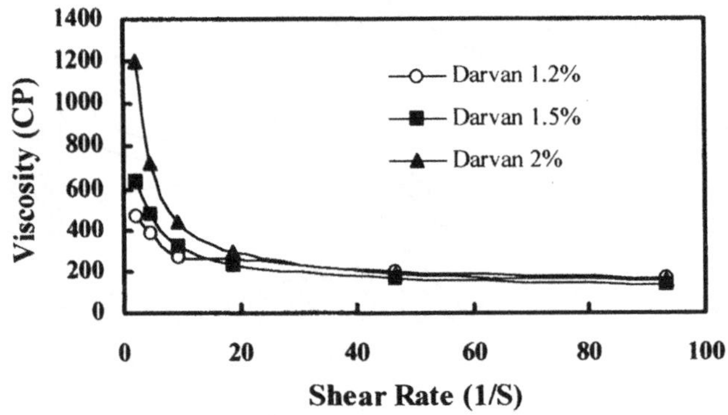

Figure 3: Effect of dispersant amount on the viscosity of ceramic slurry with 10D alumina powders.

For the present study, alumina powder, antifoaming agent and dispersant were added to water and then ball milled for 5 to 6 hours in a polyethylene bottle. The required amount of binder B-1035 (Rohm and Hass) was added to the mixture just before the infiltration. Polymeric molds, produced via FDM, were infiltrated with the ceramic slurry using a vacuum oven. The infiltrated molds were dried at room temperature for 48 to 72 hours and then subjected to binder removal and sintering cycles. Binder removal and sintering of dry ceramic powder infiltrated molds were carried out in a Thermolyne high temperature muffle furnace in furnace air environment. Samples were placed on top of a porous zirconia setter. The heating cycle that was used for the binder removal and sintering of alumina ceramics consists of three steps. During the first part of the cycle (by 350^{0}C), polymeric mold material wicks into the porous zirconia plate and then evaporates at a higher temperature (by 550^{0}C). A slower heating rate was used up to this point to avoid cracking or distortion of the part. At higher temperature, densification of alumina ceramic occurs. A final sintering temperature of 1600^{0}C and a hold time of 3 hours was used for all the samples

Porous microstructures: Figure 4a shows a schematic of the 3D honeycomb structure. Figure 4b shows the typical porous microstructures of controlled porosity alumina ceramic. Total amount of porosity can easily be varied by changing the road width and the road gap in the polymeric mold. For most of the structures, pore sizes were varied between 200 to 750 μm. Porous structures were fabricated with a continuous porous network and also structures where part of it is solid and rest of it is porous.[17]

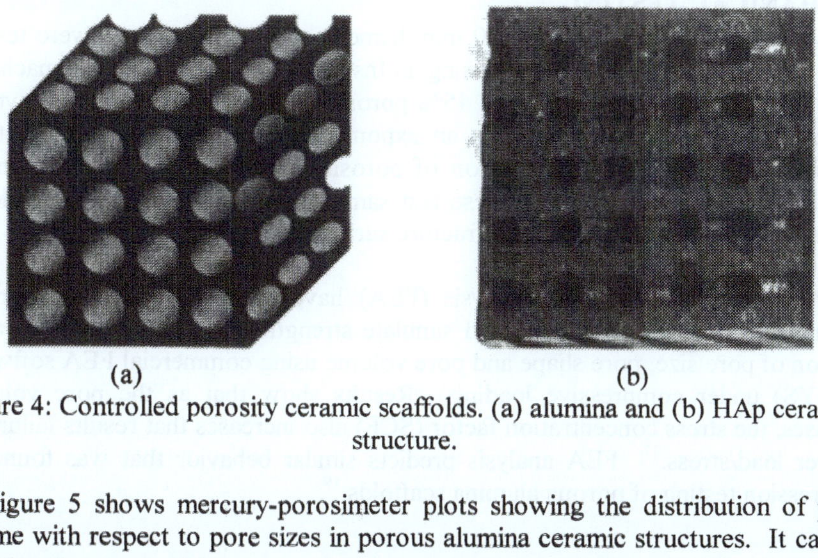

(a) (b)

Figure 4: Controlled porosity ceramic scaffolds. (a) alumina and (b) HAp ceramic structure.

Figure 5 shows mercury-porosimeter plots showing the distribution of pore volume with respect to pore sizes in porous alumina ceramic structures. It can be seen that the most of the pore volumes are concentrated between 150 to 250 μm that was the desired pore sizes for this structure. The plot also shows that keeping the pore size constant, pore volumes alone can be changed. Structures with bimodal or trimodal porosity distribution can also be fabricated by changing the starting mold design.[18] The inherent flexibility of the process can be realized from this plot.

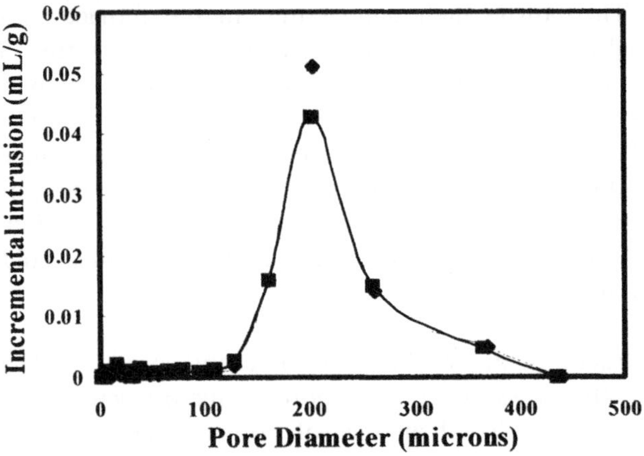

Figure 5: Hg-porosimetry plots show the variations of pore sizes in porous alumina ceramic structures

MECHANICAL TESTING

Cylindrical porous samples of 10 mm diameter and 15 mm length were tested under uniaxial compression loading using an Instron 1331 servo hydraulic machine. Initial compression data of 27% to 45% porosity alumina samples are shown in Figure 6. The failure stress shows an exponential relationship with respect to porosity, as the total volume fraction of porosity increases, the failure strength decreases. The final fracture of these test samples occurred longitudinally along the loading axis with a multifaceted fracture surface.

Preliminary finite element analysis (FEA) have been performed on porous ceramic structures to understand and simulate strength degradation behavior as a function of pore size, pore shape and pore volume using commercial FEA software (ANSYS) under compressive loading. Results show that as the pore volume increases, the stress concentration factor (SCF) also increases that results failure at a lower load/stress.[17] FEA analysis predicts similar behavior that was found in compression testing of porous alumina scaffolds.[19]

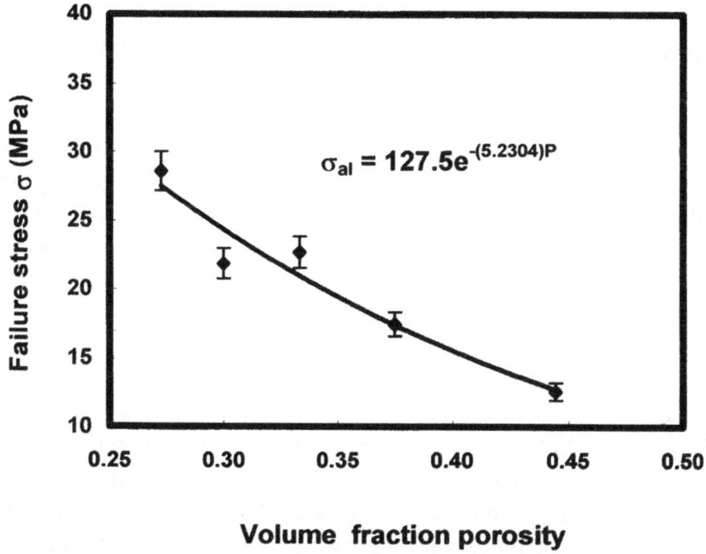

Figure 6: Effects of porosity on compression strength of porous alumina ceramics

CYTOTOXICITY AND CELL VIABILITY STUDIES

Alumina and HAp are both widely used materials that have found applications in FDA approved bone graft devices. In this process, the starting powder was non-toxic, but during processing of porous ceramic preforms, ceramic powders were mixed with different chemicals to form the structure. TGA plot for mold polymer show that less than 0.1% ash contents when fired in air environment. Binder for the ceramic slurry was selected to specifically avoid the high ash content. Once processed, all the structures were fired over 1000^0C for sintering which potentially reduces the chance of any other type of contamination. Contamination from slurry chemicals, mold polymers and ash residues after sintering are negligible but still possible.

To confirm that these porous structures are non-toxic, cytotoxicity and cell viability studies were conducted using PR1 cells (tumor cells for mice pituitary gland). Porous alumina ceramic structures and HAp coated alumina ceramic structures were used for this study. For HAp coating, HAp powders were mixed in water with anti foaming agent, dispersant and binder. The slurry was then used to coat sintered porous alumina ceramic structures. Samples were fired at 1250^0C

for 4 hours. Both porous alumina and HAp coated alumina samples were ground to form fine powders to study their cytotoxicity behavior with PR1 cells.

In Vitro cell culture (Cell viability/cytotoxicity): The PR1 cell lines were derived from a pituitary tumor of an F344 ovariectomized rat treated with estrogen for 3 months. The tumor cells were grown in culture for 28 generations and a population of cells showing PRL immunostaining and a similar shape was isolated. These cells were maintained in DMEF12 (Sigma) with 2.5% fetal calf serum (FCS, Hyclone Lab.) and 10% horse serum (HS, Hyclone Lab.) for 81-85 generations for this study.

PR1 cells were seeded on a 24 well plate at a density of 2. $5x10^5$/ ml in DMEF12 media with 2.5% FCS and 10% HS. The culture was incubated at 37^0C in humidified air with 5% CO_2 for 24 hours. The medium was replaced every two days carefully during the study. The photo was taken after 48 hours to determine the cell response towards alumina and HAp coated alumina. Cells were collected by trypsin and washed two times with the media. Then, they were resuspended in the fresh media and stained with trypan blue to count the viability for 2, 4 and 6 days. Figure 7 shows the optical micrograph of the PR1 cells on the surface of alumina after 48 hours in culture. A dense cell layer was observed in contact with both the alumina and HAp coated ceramic materials.

Figure 8 shows the cell proliferation data for 2 mg samples for 2, 4 and 6 days comparing control, alumina and HAp coated alumina samples. In general, the performance was quite comparable for both the types of ceramic materials with respect to the performance of the control samples.

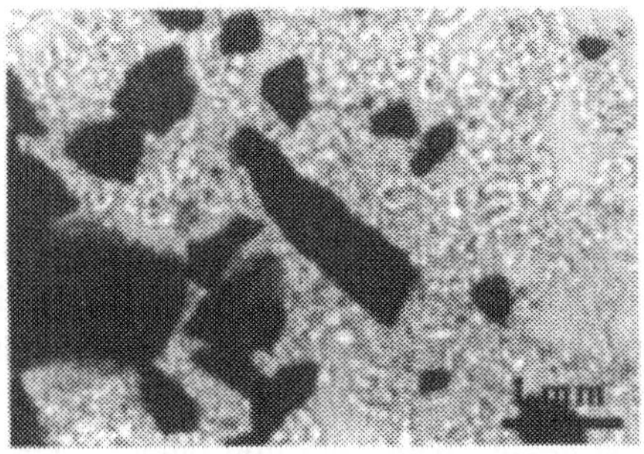

Figure 7: Optical micrograph of alumina in PR1 cells after 48 hours in culture

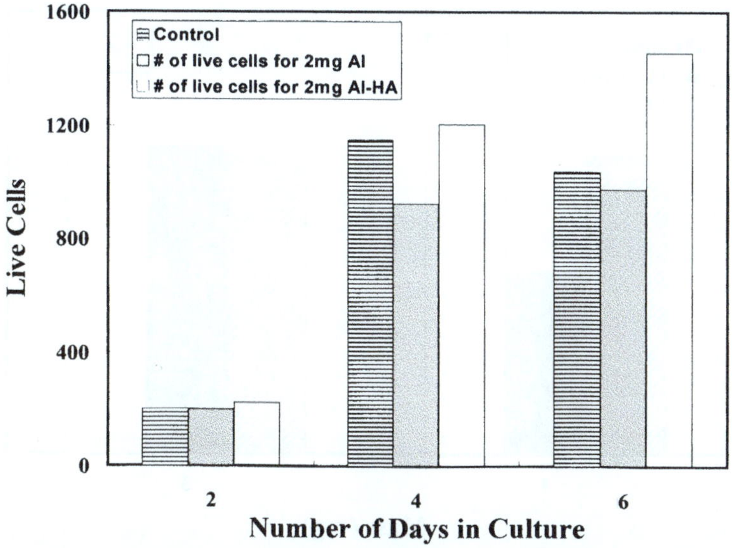

Figure 8: Cell proliferation data for 2 mg alumina and HAp coated alumina samples for 2, 4 and 6 days in culture.

Cell growth and proliferation: PR1 cells were seeded on a 24 well plate at a density of $2.5x10^5$/ml in DMEF12 media with 2.5% FCS and 10%HS. The culture was incubated at 37^0C in humidified air with 5% CO_2 for 24 hours. Pre-weighed alumina and HAp coated alumina was added in each well. Adding 40 μl Cell Titer 96 Aqueous One Solution Reagent (Promega) into each well of the 24 well assay plate containing the samples in 200 μl of culture medium. The plates were incubated for 3-4 hours at 37^0C in a humidified 5% CO_2 atmosphere. Final record of the UV absorbance was taken at 490 nm using a 96 well plate reader. Figure 9 shows the plot of absorbance vs. the initial wieght of alumina and HAp coated alumina materials after 2 days in culture.

Weight change in porous samples: 1 cm long and 2 mm in diameter cylindrical porous pre-weighed alumina samples were immersed in 1.5 ml of DMEF12 media and the changes in weight were measured in the time interval of 3, 7, 14 and 21 days. Initially an increase in weight was found after 3 days, which may be due to the salt deposition on the porous scaffolds. A continuous increase in weight was also found with rest of the samples after 7, 14 and 21 days. Figure 10 shows a bar chart for the weight change of porous alumina samples with respect to the number of days in culture.

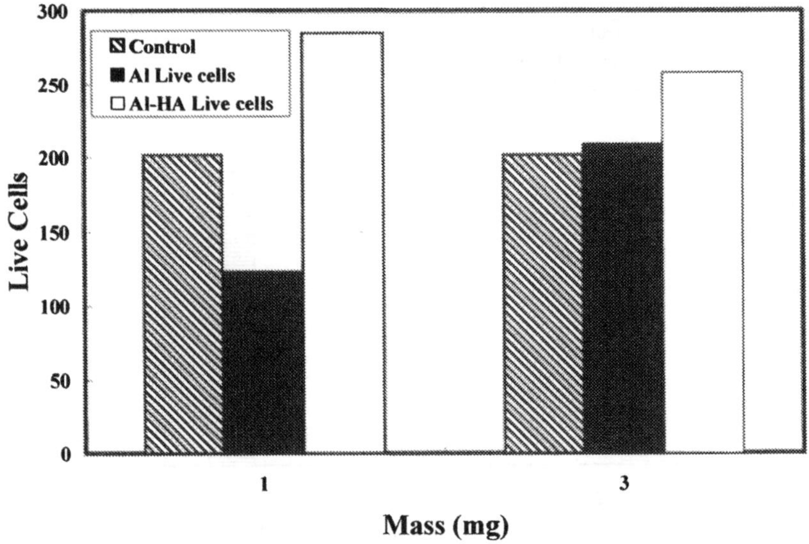

Figure 9: Absorbance plot shows the relative cell proliferation of control, alumina and HAp coated alumina samples

CONCLUSIONS

Porous alumina ceramics have been fabricated with different porosity (20-50 percent by volume) by controlling the pore size (a, z_{gap}) and pore spacing (x_{gap}, y_{gap}) using indirect FDM process. The pore sizes were varied between 200 to 750 μm. Initial uniaxial compression tests show that the increasing the amount of porosity decreases the strength of porous alumina ceramic materials. It was found that the alumina and HAp coated-alumina provide favorable sites for cell attachment for PR1 cells which reveals that these composites may favor bone bonding when implanted *in vivo*. Both the cytotoxicity and cell proliferation data showed that there was no contamination due to processing of these porous ceramic implants.

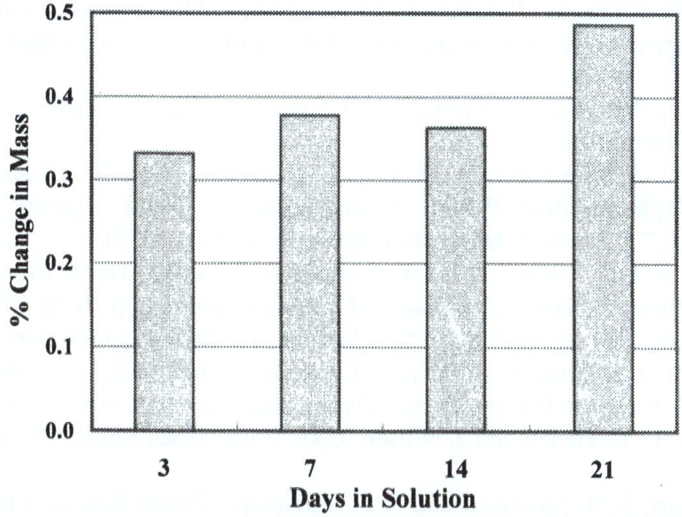

Figure 10: % change in weight for porous alumina ceramics in DMEF12 media

ACKNOWLEDGEMENTS

Authors would like to acknowledge National Science Foundation for the financial support through NSF-CAREER program (DMI-9874971). Experimental support by Raj Atisivan and Ashwin Hattiangadi is also acknowledged. Authors would also like to thank Dr. N. K. Vail of Kestrel Medica Inc. for useful discussions.

REFERENCES

1. a) L. L. Hench and J. Wilson, "An Introduction to Bioceramics," World Scientific, London, U.K. (1993). b) L. L. Hench, "Bioceramics," J. Am. Ceram.Soc. 81(7), 1705-28 (1998).
2. S. F. Hulbert, J. C. Bokros, L. L. Hench, J. Wilson and G. Heimke, "Ceramics in Clinical Applications: Past, Present and Future"; pp 189-213 in High Tech Ceramics. Edited by P.Vincenzini, Elsvier, Amsterdam, The Netherlands, (1987).
3. L. L. Hench and E. C. Ethridge, "Biomaterials: An Interfacial approach," Academic Press, New York, (1982).
4. A. Ravaglioli and A. Krajewski, "Bioceramics: Materials, Properties, Applications," Chapman and Hall, London (1992).

5. U. Gross, R. Kinne, H. J. Schmitz and V. Strunz, "The response of Bone to Surface Active Glass/Glass-Ceramics," CRC Crit. Rev. Biocompat., 4, 2, (1988).
6. L. L. Hench, "Bioceramics: From Concepts to Clinic," J. Am. Ceram. Soc., 74 [7], 1487-510 (1991).
7. E. W. White, J. N. Webber, D. M. Roy, E. L. Owen, R. T. Chiroff and R. A. White, "Replamineform Porous Biomaterials for Hard Tissue Implant Applications," *J. Biomed. Mater. Res. Symp.*, **6**, p 23-7 (1975).
8. R. T. Chiroff, E. W. White, J. N. Webber and D. M. Roy, "Tissue Ingrowth of Replamineform Implants," *J. Biomed. Mater. Res. Symp.*, **6**, p 29-45 (1975).
9. A. F. Tencer, and E. C. Shors, "Mechanical and Biological Properties of a Porous Polymer-Coated Caralline Ceramic," Handbook of Bioactive CeramicsII: Calcium Phosphate and Hydroxylapatite Ceramics, edited by T. Yamamura, L. L. Hench and J. Wilson, CRC Press, Boca Raton, FL, pp 209-21 (1990).
10. S. F. Hulbert, S. J. Morrison and J. J. Klawitter, "Tissue Reaction to Three Ceramics of Porous and Non-Porous Structures," *J. Biomed. Mater. Res. Symp.*, **6**, p 347-74 (1975).
11. S. F. Hulbert, J. R. Matthews, J. J. Klawitter, B. W. Sauer and R. B. Leonard, "Effect of Stress on Tissue Ingrowth into Porous Aluminum Oxide," *J. Biomed. Mater. Res. Symp.*, **5**, p 85-97 (1974).
12. C. P. A. T. Klein, and P. Patka, "A Comparison Between HA and Whitlockite Macroporous Ceramics Implanted in Dog Femurs," Handbook of Bioactive CeramicsII: Calcium Phosphate and Hydroxylapatite Ceramics, edited by T. Yamamura, L. L. Hench and J. Wilson, CRC Press, Boca Raton, FL, pp 53-60 (1990).
13. James, W.J., M.A. Slabbekoorn, W.A. Edgin, and C.K. Hardin, "Correction of Congenital Malar Hypoplasia Using Stereolithography for Presurgical Planning," *J. Oral Maxillofac. Surg.*, **56**, 512-517, 1998.
14. Holle, J., K. Vinzenz, E. Würinger, K.-J. Kulenkampff, and M. Saidi, "The Prefabricated Combined Scapula Flap for Bony and Soft-Tissue Reconstruction in Maxillofacial Defects – A New Method", *Plastic and Reconstructive Surgery*, **98** [3], 542-552 (1996).
15. Erickson, D., Lt. Col., D.D.S., M.S., MacKown Dental Laboratory, Lackland Air Force Base, San Antonio, Texas, *personal communication*, 1997.
16. "Rapid Prototyping Using FDM: A Fast, Precise, Safe Technology," pp. 301-308 in Solid Freeform Fabrication Proceedings (Austin, TX, August 1992). Edited by, H. L. Marcus, J. J. Beamen, J. W. Barlow, D L. Bourell, and R. H. Crawford. University of Texas at Austin, 1992.

17. Bose, S. M. Avila, and A. Bandyopadhyay, "Processing of Bioceramic Implants via Fused Deposition Process," Solid Freeform Fabrication Symposium Proceedings, **9**, 629-436 (1998).
18. Bose, S., Bandyopadhyay, A., *unpublished data*, Washington State University, 1999.
19. A. Hattiangadi, R. Atisivan, S. Bose and A. Bandyopadhyay, "Strength Degradation in Controlled Porosity Ceramic Structures Under Compressive Loading," submitted for publication to the Journal of the American Ceramic Society, March 1999.

DEVELOPMENT OF BIOCERAMIC TISSUE SCAFFOLDS VIA FUSED DEPOSITION OF CERAMICS

Iván A. Cornejo, Thomas F. McNulty, Shelliam Lee, Ernest Bianchi, Stephen C. Danforth and Ahmad Safari
Department of Ceramic and Materials Engineering, Rutgers University
607 Taylor Road
Piscataway, NJ 08854-8065

Kevor S. TenHuisen and Victor F. Janas
J&J Corporate Biomaterials Center, a Division of Ethicon Inc.
Rt. 22 West, P.O. Box 151
Somerville, NJ 08876-0151

ABSTRACT

Solid freeform fabrication (SFF) is one of the fastest growing fields in the general area of manufacturing. SFF is a generic term for novel prototyping/manufacturing techniques for making structures, without the help of hard tooling, dies, or molds, from a computer-aided design (CAD) data portrait of the desired structure. Hence, SFF techniques provide ways for making a variety of complex shaped structures that are difficult, costly, or simply impossible to manufacture by conventional techniques.

In this research, Fused Deposition of Ceramics (FDC), developed at Rutgers University, was utilized to fabricate a variety of novel structures with controlled macrostructure (pore size and distribution, connectivity, tortuosity and orientation) for tissue scaffolding applications. The design, fabrication, physical and mechanical properties and critical issues in processing these novel structures will be discussed in this article.

INTRODUCTION

Biomaterials are expected to have an increasing role in healthcare in the next century. In addition, bioceramics are expected to play a major role in hard tissue replacement in the near future. Today, there is an increasing need for bone replacements in humans due to accidents, birth defects, hereditary disorders, conditions, and diseases. Endogenous or exogenous bone can replace the damaged or lost bone tissue. However, the use of an endogenous bone substance involves additional surgery and is available in limited quantities. Furthermore, implant rejection and/or transmission of diseases are the major disadvantages of exogenous bone implants. On the other hand, metals have been widely used for load bearing applications. However, metals are not ideal materials since corrosion, tissue sensitization, wear and stress shielding can all occur with metal implants.

Tissue scaffolding ceramics derived from calcium phosphates, such as hydroxyapatite (HAp, $Ca_{10}(PO_4)_6(OH)_2$) and β-tricalcium phosphate (TCP, $Ca_3(PO_4)_2$), have been used as synthetic bone substitutes [1]. When used as a bone fillers, porous bioceramic structures made of HAp and TCP (100-500 μm pore size) have been found to be osteoconductive, allowing for the growth of hard and soft bone tissue into and around the scaffold. Porous scaffolds allow the bone tissue to grow into the pores, increasing the strength of the implant. However, the minimum pore size required to enable ingrowth of the surrounding bone together with blood supply is about 100 μm. This requirement together with the uncontrolled and non-uniform pore sizes and distributions (in current scaffolds produced by classical fabrication techniques) decreases the strength of the implants significantly, resulting in very poor mechanical properties of the implant and limits their usage to non-load bearing applications [1-5]. In addition, the lack of methodologies for the preparation of calcium phosphate powders with controlled physical and chemical characteristics, and the lack of sufficient knowledge about the type of calcium phosphate deemed optimum for bioimplantation, have limited the usage of these materials.

Solid freeform fabrication (SFF) is one of the fastest growing fields in the general area of manufacturing [6]. At Rutgers University, SFF techniques have been developed to fabricate novel and complex structures using a variety of materials, including piezoelectrics, relaxors, bio- and structural ceramics, metals, and plastics for sensor, medical imaging, non-destructive testing, actuator, medical applications, etc. (Figure 1). SFF is a family of novel prototyping / manufacturing techniques for making structures without the help of any hard tooling dies or molds. All SFF techniques begin with a common approach, namely, a computer-aided design (CAD) data portrait of the desired structure. Using the CAD file as input, the final part is deposited layer by layer on a platform. The depositing fixture moves along x and y directions while the platform moves along the z direction (Figure 2). Hence, the SFF techniques provide ways for making a variety of complex shaped structures that are difficult, costly or simply impossible to manufacture by conventional techniques.

In this research, Fused Deposition of Ceramics (FDC), developed at Rutgers University [7-9], was utilized to fabricate a variety of novel structures for porous tissue scaffolding and orthopedic devices [10] with controlled macrostructures for bone prosthesis (pore size and distribution, connectivity and orientation). The

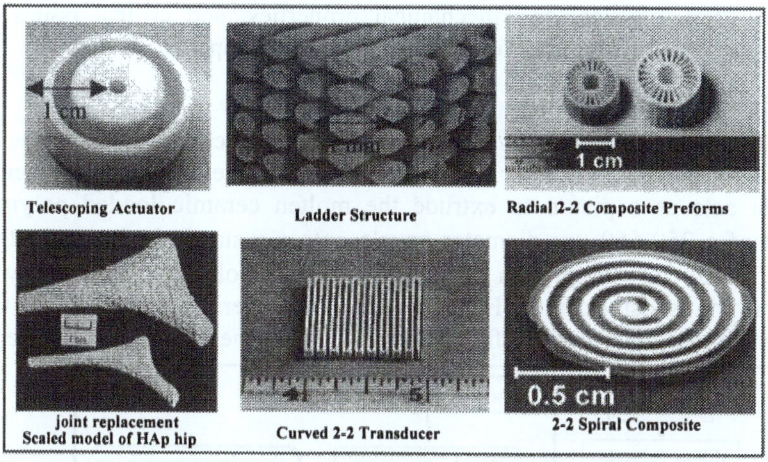

Figure 1. Novel ceramic and composite structures fabricated by FDC. This mosaic of pictures shows the potential of FDC manufacture in different areas of today's technology.

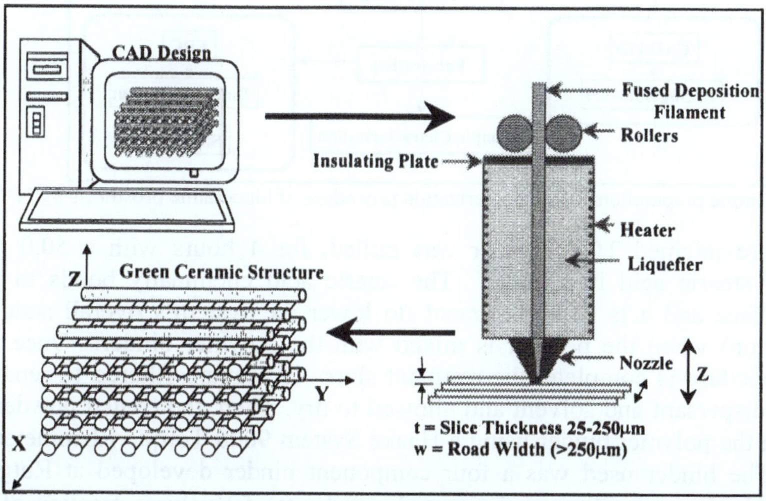

Figure 2. Fused Deposition of Ceramics (FDC) process. A CAD file of the desired part is input to the computer. The final part is then deposited layer by layer in a movable platform.

design, fabrication, physical and mechanical properties, and critical issues in processing these novel structures will be discussed in this paper.

EXPERIMENTAL PROCEDURE

The first step in making any structure by the FDC technique is to fabricate the feedstock filament (ceramic or metal particle loaded thermoplastic filament). The filament acts as a piston to extrude the molten ceramic loaded polymer material out of a 250-650 μm diameter nozzle onto a z-stage platform. In this research, a 52 vol. % β-tricalcium phosphate* (TCP) / polymer compound was made to act as the feedstock in the FDC process. The generic processing for TCP parts from particle loaded filament fabrication is shown schematically in Figure 3.

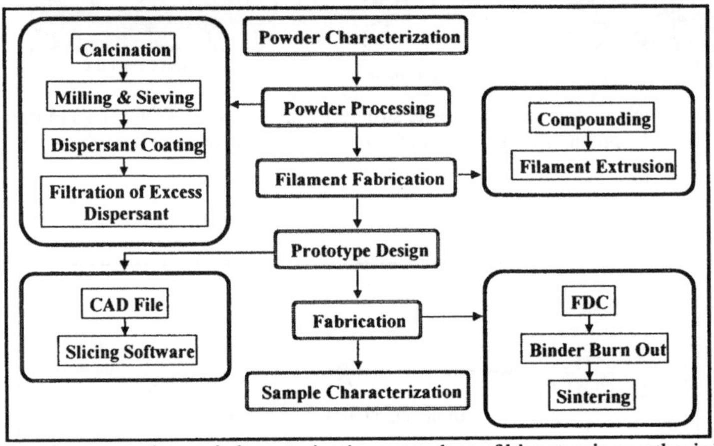

Figure 3. Sample preparation and characterization procedure of bioceramic prosthesis by FDC.

First, the pre-calcined TCP powder was milled, for 4 hours with a 50.0 g/L solution of stearic acid in toluene. The stearic acid chemically bonds to the powder surface and acts as a dispersant (to lower the system's overall state of agglomeration) when the powder is mixed with the polymer binder. Once the coating procedure is complete, the resultant slurry is vacuum filtered to remove the excess dispersant and solvent and allowed to dry. Then, the coated powder is mixed with the polymer binder using a Haake System 9000 Torque Rheometer at 100 rpm. The binder used was a four component binder developed at Rutgers (ECG9) [11]. Compounding of the coated powder (to 52-volume fraction of β-TCP ceramic) with binder was carried out in a 45 cc mixing bowl heated between 140 and 160°C for a total time of 70 minutes. The compounded material is then granulated into mm-sized pebbles and extruded in the form of filaments with close control over their diameter (1.78 ± 0.01 mm) using an Instron™ Model

* β-$Ca_3(PO_4)_2$, Cam Implants bv, The Netherlands

4505 mechanical testing unit with a capillary extrusion attachment. Extrusion was carried out at 85-90°C at a feed rate of 1.0 mm/min. Each filament was then cut to a 30-cm length.

The next step was to create a CAD file** of the desired bio-structure (.stl file). Quickslice software (Stratasys, Inc.) was then utilized to slice the CAD file and to create the tool path (.slc file). Once the tool-path was created, the file was saved as machine readable .sml file and sent to a modified Stratasys 3-D Modeler^{TM}. The nozzle diameter, slice thickness and road width were selected to be 300, 250 and 350 μm respectively. The FDC build parameters such as: liquefier temperature, envelope temperature, flow rate, start delay, pre-flow, start flow, start distance, main flow, shutoff distance, roll back, speed and acceleration of the nozzle during deposition, were modified for part quality. Table I shows the modified flow parameters and their default values.

Table I. Flow Parameters and their Values for ICW04 (Default) and ECG9 / 52 vol. % TCP (Modified).

Parameters	Default values	Modified values
Start delay (sec)	0.106	0.1
Pre-flow	27	33
Start flow	21	18
Start distance (mm)	0.69	0.69
Main flow	122	122
Shutoff distance (mm)	0.53	0.53
Roll back	169	169
Speed (mm/s)	20.3	7.62
Liquefier Temperature (°C)	67-70	165
Envelope Temperature (°C)	35	30

The green β-TCP structures made by the FDC process were subjected to binder burnout (BBO) cycle and sintering heat treatments to consolidate the structures. Since the parts had fine features, the BBO cycle was optimized to maintain part integrity. The BBO cycle was chosen based on a TGA/DTA analysis of the filaments used (Figure 4). The BBO profile used was set as follows: room temperature (RT) to 175°C at 300°C/h, 175 to 500°C at 5°C/h with 4 hours dwell time at 500°C, and from 500 to RT at 300°C/h. Sintering was carried out in a box furnace under static air atmosphere conditions. In this firing cycle, the FDC parts were placed on a TCP powder bed inside an alumina crucible with cover. The furnace was first heated at 210°C/h from RT to 1000°C.

** Pro/Engineer, Parametric Technology Corporation, Waltham, MA

Then, the heating rate was reduced to 60°C/h to reach the sintering temperature*** of 1250°C with a dwell time of 1 hour. Finally, the furnace was allowed to cool to RT at a rate of 300°C/h.

The as-received and calcined powders, as well as the sintered structures, were characterized by scanning electron microscopy (SEM), field emission SEM (FESEM), x-ray diffraction (XRD), density measurements [12], chemical analysis [13], and 4-point bending measurements [14].

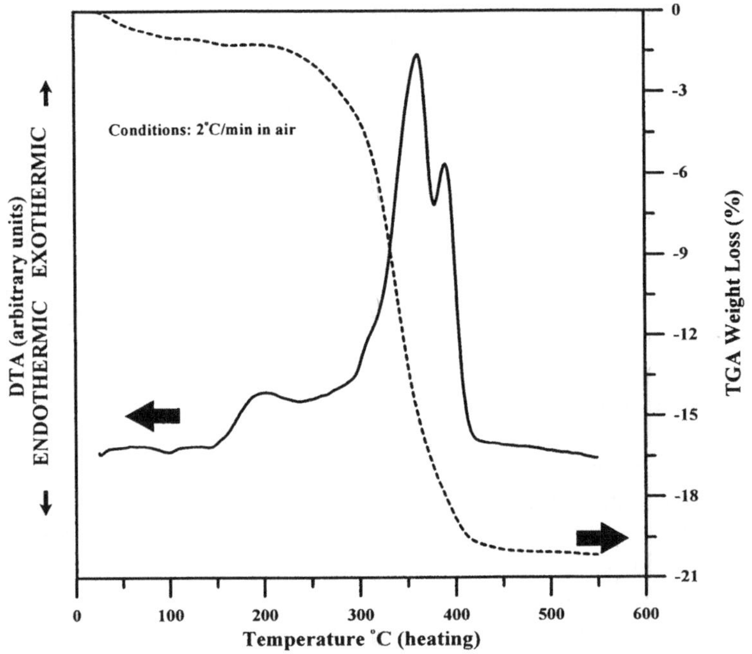

Figure 4. DTA (solid line) and TGA (dashed line) profiles of 52 vol. % TCP / ECG9 filaments extruded through a 300 μm nozzle.

RESULTS AND DISCUSSION

The powder characteristics, including particle size, particle size distribution, surface area, and state of agglomeration play an important role in the rheological and mechanical properties of the feedstock filament. The BET surface area of the as-received powders was found to be 37.41 m^2/g, which corresponds to a mean particle size of 0.056 μm (assuming spherical monosized particles). However, the state of agglomeration was found to be high and large agglomerates were found to

*** See RESULTS & DISCUSSION Section for more details about the calcination and sintering temperatures.

be present in the as-received powders, as shown in the FESEM micrographs shown in Figure 5a. Furthermore, the as-received powders were bi-phasic, and the major phase detected by XRD did not corresponded to the desired β-TCP phase (see bottom curve in Figure 6). The as-received powders were calcined at different temperatures and times to decrease the surface area and thus reduce the state of agglomeration of the powders. Calcination was also performed to form the β-TCP phase. Table II shows the physical characteristic of the calcined powders. From Figure 6, it can be seen that these powders transform to pure β-TCP after calcination of the powders at 925°C. It was found that the BET surface area of these powders decreased to 3.38 m^2/g which correspond to a mean particle size of 0.58 μm (see Table II). SEM and FESEM studies revealed that the powders consisted mostly of agglomerates and upon calcination the agglomerate size shrunk, forming thin necks between particles (Figure 5). Based on these results, it was decided to calcine the as-received powders at 925°C for 1 hour followed by a short ball-milling step of 4 hours to break up the soft agglomerates. Sieving the calcined and milled powder through a mesh size of 150 μm (100 mesh) before coating the powders was necessary.

Table II. TCP Powder Characteristics after Calcination at Different Temperatures and Times.

Calcination Cycle		Surface Area (m^2/g)	Powder Density (g/cm^3)	Particle Size (μm)
Temperature (°C)	Time (h)			
RT	None	37.41	2.87	0.056
800	1	13.10	--	--
800	2	11.00	--	--
850	2	9.293	--	--
900	1	6.502	3.066	0.301
925	1	3.380	3.060	0.580
925	2	2.570	--	--
925	3	4.296	3.044	0.459

In the initial stages of this research, the FDC parts were made from pure β-TCP powders. However, TCP undergoes a phase transformation from β- to α-phase at 1180°C [15], limiting the sintering temperature of the parts to 1150°C. Pressed TCP samples sintered at 1150°C reached a density of 2.71 g/cm^3, which is only 88.6% of the theoretical density. When the sintering temperature was elevated to 1250°C, the density was reduced to 2.44 g/cm^3 due to the α-β phase transformation (Table III). To increase the sintering temperature and suppress the α-phase formation, the as-received TCP powders were doped with 5 mole % of $Mg_3(PO_4)_2$. Small additions of $Mg_3(PO_4)_2$ have been found to extend the β-phase

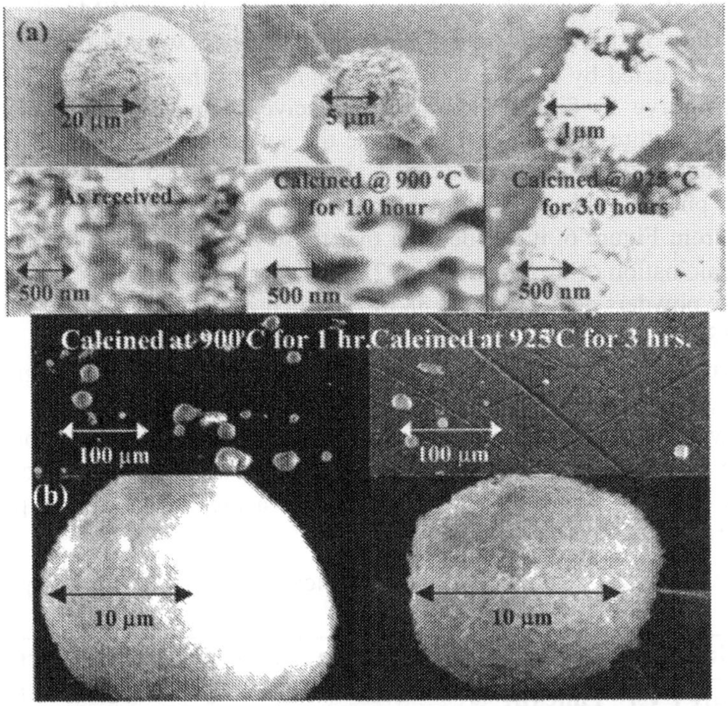

Figure 5. FESEM (a) and SEM (b) of the as-received and calcined powders of TCP show the degree and evolution of agglomerates after heat treatment.

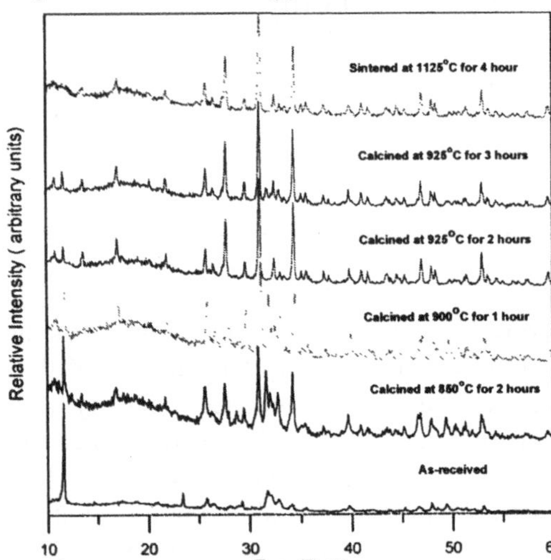

Figure 6. XRD patterns of pure as-received TCP and powders calcined at different temperatures and times. The tick marks at the bottom correspond to the JCPDS file of ß-TCP.

stability to above 1400°C [15]. Density measurements on doped TCP samples (M-TCP) are compared with un-doped samples (TCP) in Table III. As can be seen from this Table, there are no changes in the density values of TCP and M-TCP pressed samples when sintered at 1150°C. However, when the sintering temperature was elevated to 1250°C, the improvement in the density data is remarkable for both pressed and FDC samples.

Table III. Density Measurements (given in g/cm^3) on Pressed and FDC Sintered Samples (for 1 hour). The Percent of the Theoretical Density is Given in Parenthesis.

Temperature (°C)	**TCP Pressed Pellets**	**M-TCP Pressed Pellets**	**M-TCP FDC Bars**
1150	2.71 ± 0.04 (88.6)	2.69 ± 0.07 (87.9)	--
1250	2.44 ± 0.04 (79.7)	2.99 ± 0.02 (97.7)	3.05 ± 0.03 (99.7)

Figure 7 shows the powder XRD patterns of TCP and M-TCP samples heat-treated at different temperatures and times. Notice that all the samples have similar XRD profiles. These patterns were identical to the JCPDS files for β-TCP [16] (within the experimental resolution), and no significant changes in the peak intensity were observed. These results indicated that the β-TCP phase was stabilized with the $Mg_3(PO_4)_2$ doping. Furthermore, the M-TCP samples reached a theoretical density of 97.7 and 99.7 % in both pressed and FDC samples (Table III) when sintered at 1250°C.

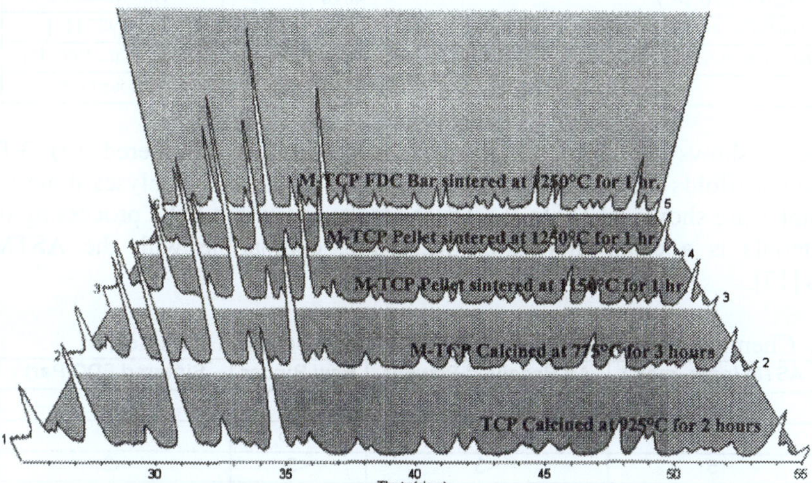

Figure 7. XRD profiles of TCP and M-TCP powders and parts heat-treated at different temperatures and times. All the peaks match the JCPDS files of β-TCP.

Figure 8 shows a green, four-point bend mechanical test bar fabricated by FDC. After sintering and machining to the ASTM B-type standard dimensions [14], the bars were broken and the four-point bending strength calculated. Table IV shows the preliminary results obtained. The results approach those of the published data, however, further research is necessary to improve the strength, reduce warping during sintering, and study other mechanical and biological properties.

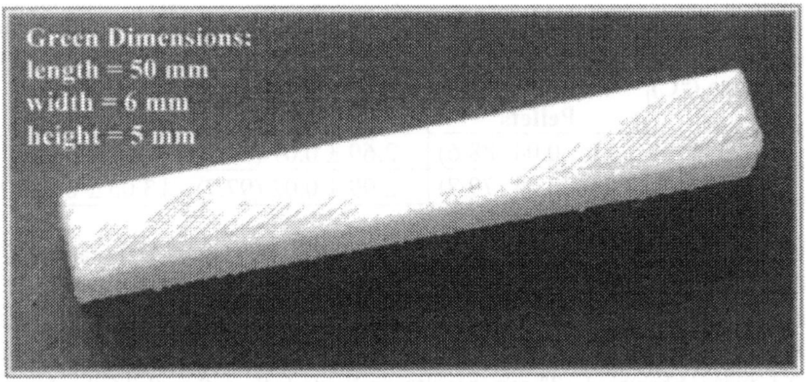

Figure 8. Four-point bend mechanical test specimen (ASTM type B) fabricated by FDC (green).

Table IV. Mechanical Properties of Calcium Phosphates.

Materials (Method)	Bending Strength (MPa)	Source
$Ca_3(PO_4)_2 + Mg_3(PO_4)_2$ (FDC)	40±8	This Research
$Ca_3(PO_4)_2 + Na_5P_3O_{10}$ in H_2O (isostatic compaction)	25-30	Hon, 1987 [17]
$(NH_4)_2(HPO_4) + Ca(NO_3)_2$	45-50	Royer et al., 1993 [5]
Bone	120-235	Various [1-3]

Figure 9 shows an isometric view of green (a) and sintered (b) 3-D honeycomb scaffolds for bone replacement studies. Chemical analyses done on these samples are shown in Table V. These results show that FDC processing of TCP materials is a clean fabrication technique, compatible with the ASTM standards [13].

Table V. Chemical Analysis Results of FDC Porous Scaffold Samples.

Impurity	ASTM (ppm, max.)	As Received Powder	Raw Binder	Sintered FDC Part
Pb	30	<5	5	10
Hg	5	<0.5	<0.5	--
Cd	5	<3	<3	<2

Figure 10 shows an isometric view of an orthopedic device developed for J&J Corporation. The device consists of a biocompatible hollow wedge having upper and lower porous surfaces. These surfaces are spanned by reinforcing elements or pillars to increase the mechanical strength of the device. Notice that the complexity of the structure impedes the manufacture by conventional ceramic processing techniques.

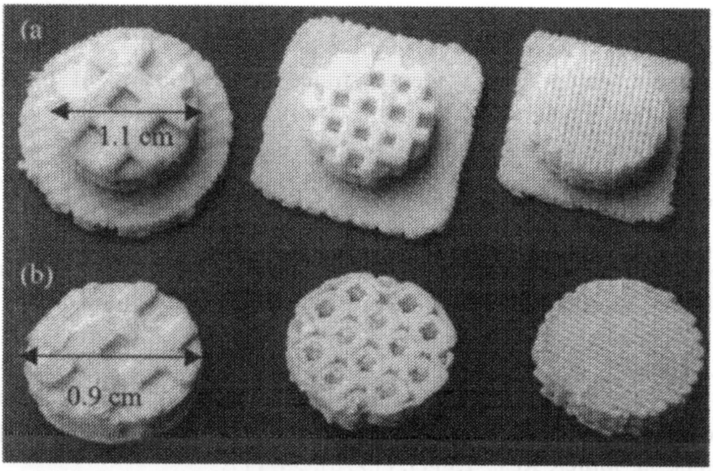

Figure 9. Porous Scaffolds built in a stacking layer ABABAB configuration by FDC. (a) Green FDC scaffolds. The road width was from left to right 1.26, 0.56, and 0.20 mm, respectively. The gap width was from left to right 1.90, 1.20, and 0.30 mm, respectively. (b) Sintered FDC Scaffolds.

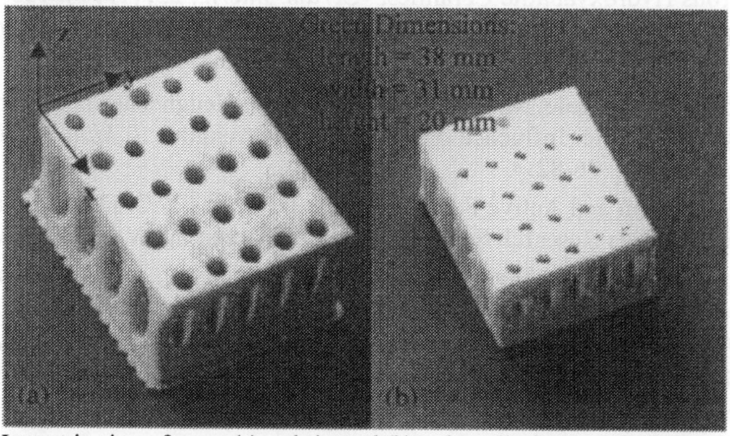

Figure 10. Isometric view of green (a) and sintered (b) orthopedic device manufactured by FDC. The structure consists of interconnected channels of different geometry and dimensions. The overall shrinkage was found to be 16, 18, and 18% in the x, y, and z directions, respectively.

SUMMARY AND CONCLUSIONS

Different scaffolds and orthopedic devices were successfully made by the FDC technique. Four-point bend testing bars were fabricated by FDC and mechanically tested. The results, although preliminary, are similar with those found in published literature. Chemical analysis on FDC products showed that the FDC process is a clean manufacturing process and met the ASTM criteria.

This research program has demonstrated the feasibility of manufacturing scaffold and orthopedic devices with controlled dimensional tolerances and features by the FDC technique.

ACKNOWLEDGEMENTS

This work was financially supported by The Johnson & Johnson Corporate Biomaterials Center. The author would like to thank Dr. R. Panda and Mr. P. Teung for their helpful comments and critics during the evolution of this project.

REFERENCES

1. W. Suchanek and M. Yoshimura, "Processing and Properties of Hydroxyapatite-Based Biomaterials for Use as Hard Tissue Replacement Implants," *J. Mater. Res.,* **13** [1], (1998): 94-117.
2. L.L. Hench, "Bioceramics," *J. Am. Ceram. Soc.,* **81** [7], (1998): 1705-28.
3. D. M Liu, "Influence of Porosity and Pore Size on the Compressive Strength of Porous Hydroxyapatite Ceramics," *Ceram. Intern.,* **23,** (1997): 135-9.
4. D. M Liu, "Porous Hydroxyapatite Ceramics," *Key Engineering Materials,* **115,** (1996): 209-32.
5. A. Royer, J.C. Viguie, M. Heughebaert, and J.C. Heughebaert, "Stoichiometry of Hydroxyapatite: Influence on the Flexural Strength", *J. Mater. Sci. Mater. Med.,* **4,** (1993): 76-82.
6. Solid Freeform and Active Fabrication, ed. D. Dimos, S.C. Danforth, and M.J. Cima, Materials Research Soc., Symposium Proceedings Vol. 542, PA (1999).
7. S.C. Danforth, M. Agarwala, A. Bandyopadghyay, N. Langrana, V.R. Jamalabad, A. Safari, and R. van Weeren, US Patent No. 5,738,817 (1998).
8. A. Bandyopadhyay, R.K. Panda, T.F. McNulty, F. Mohammadi, S.C. Danforth, and A. Safari, "Piezoelectric Ceramics and Composites Via Rapid Prototyping Techniques," *Rapid Prototyping,* **4** [1] (1998): 37-49.
9. S.C. Danforth, M. Jafari, and N. Langrana, "Solid Freeform Fabrication of Functional Advanced Ceramic Components," *Naval Research Reviews,* **L** [3] (1998): 27-38.
10. V.F. Janas and K. TenHuisen, Private Communication (1998).

11. T.F. McNulty, F. Mohammadi, A. Bandyopadhyay, D.J. Shanefield, S.C. Danforth, and A. Safari, "Development of a Binder Formulation for Fused Deposition of Ceramics," *Rapid Prototyping*, **4** [4], (1998): 144-50.

12. ASTM Designation: C 373-56, "Standard Method of Test for Water Adsorption, Bulk Density, Apparent Porosity and Apparent Specific Gravity of Fired Porous Whiteware Products".

13. ASTM Designation: F 1088-87, "Standard Specification for Beta-Tricalcium Phosphate for Surgical Implantation".

14. ASTM Designation: C 1161-90, "Standard Test Method for Flexural Strength of Advanced Ceramics at Ambient Temperature".

15. Phase Diagrams for Ceramists, ed. E.M. Levin, Am. Ceram. Soc., OH (1964): 214.

16. JCPDS X-ray Diffraction Card Number 09-0169.

17. M. Hon and F. Lin, "A Study of the Sintering of β-Tricalciumphosphate Bioceramics", *High Tech Ceramics* (1987).

KEYWORD AND AUTHOR INDEX

Alumina, 67, 167

Bandyopadhyay, Amit, 167
Bayraktar, Defne, 39
Beta-tricalcium phosphate, 183
Bianchi, Ernest, 183
Bioactivity, 15
Bioceramics, 103, 167, 183
Bioglass®, 1
Bioimplant material, 53
Biomimetics, 39, 81
Bioresorbable, 113
Body fluids, 39
Bone, 1
    prosthesis, 183
Borum, L., 93
Bose, Susmita, 167

Calcium phosphate, 157
Carbonated, 39
Case, E.D., 53
Castkova, K., 157
Cell carriers, 67
Characterization, 145
Cihlar, J., 157
Clare, A.G., 113
Coatings, 15, 145, 157
Cochlear implant, 129
Cornejo, Iván A., 183
Crimp, Melissa J., 1

Danforth, Stephen C., 183
Darsell, Jens, 167
Density, 25
Dickens, E., 93
Dissolution, 113
Doctor, Udhav U., 1

Eckert, K.-L., 67
Electrophoretic mobility, 93
Enameling, 15
Enzyme urease, 39
Esposito, L., 103

Fibers, 113
Friedrich, H., 81
Fu, L., 145
Fused deposition, 183

Gadow, R., 67
Glass, 15, 113
Glass fibers, 113
Gomez-Vega, J.M., 15
Greil, P., 81

Hardness, 25
Hierarchial microstructure, 81
High-energy milling, 25
Hip joint prosthesis, 103
Hoepfner, T.P., 53
Hydroxyapatite, 1, 15, 25, 39, 53, 145, 167

In vitro, 113, 129
Infiltration, 157

Janas, Victor F., 183
Jaworski, A., 93
Jez, M., 157

Kaindl, A., 81
Khor, K.A., 145

Layered double hydroxide, 93
Lee, S.H., 113
Lee, Shelliam, 183
Lim, V.J.P., 145

Marshall, G.W., 15
Marshall, S.J., 15
McNulty, Thomas F., 183
Mechanical activation, 25
Mechanical properties, 157
Microcracks, 53
Mukherjee, N., 129

Nanocomposites, 93
Ng, S.C., 25

Olorunyolemi, T., 93
Oppermann, Dean A., 1
Oriakhi, C., 93
Oxide ceramics, 157

Piezoelectrics, 129
Plasma spraying, 145
Polymer adsorption, 93
Porous structures, 167
Porous tissue scaffolds, 183
PR1 cells, 167
Pressure casting, 103
PZT, 129

Roseman, R.D., 129

Safari, Ahmad, 183
Saiz, E., 15
Salomoni, A., 103
Sarkar, Dipak K., 167
Sieber, H., 81
Silicon carbide, 81
Solid freeform fabrication, 167, 183
Spray drying, 67
Stamenkovic, I., 103

Tas, A. Cüneyt, 39
TenHuisen, Kevor S., 183
Thermal expansion, 53
Ti-6AL-4V, 15
Tissue engineering, 183
Titania, 67
Tomsia, A.P., 15
Trunec, M., 157
Tucci, A., 103

Urea, 39

Wang, J., 25
Willging, J.P., 129
Wilson, O.C., Jr., 93
Wintermantel, E., 67
Woodlike cearmics, 81

Yang, Lihua, 167
Yeong, K.C.B., 25
Young, D., 93

Zirconia, 145
 -alumina, 103

Printed and bound by CPI Group (UK) Ltd, Croydon, CR0 4YY
15/09/2026
14962409-0001